Communicati

Development

Profile

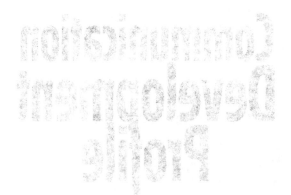

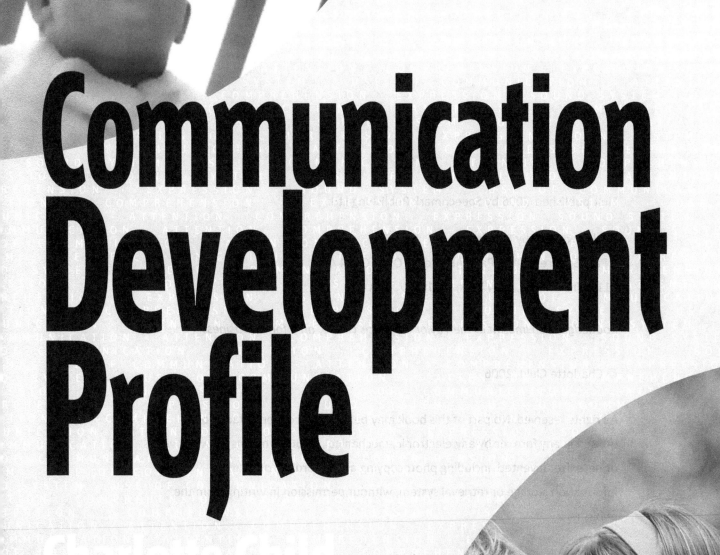

Communication Development Profile

Charlotte Child

Routledge
Taylor & Francis Group

LONDON AND NEW YORK

Dedication

For my daughters, Agatha, Verity and Florence, who brought my work to life, and for my husband, Nick, and the wonderful sound of the wine being opened.

For the purposes of clarity alone, throughout this text 'he' is used to refer to the child.

First published 2006 by Speechmark Publishing Ltd.

Published 2017 by Routledge

2 Park Square, Milton Park, Abingdon, Oxon OX14 4RN

711 Third Avenue, New York, NY 10017, USA

Routledge is an imprint of the Taylor & Francis Group, an informa business

© Charlotte Child, 2006

British Library Cataloguing in Publication Data
Child, Charlotte
      Communication development profile
      1. Communication disorders in children 2. Medical records I. Title
      618.9'2855075

ISBN 978 0 86388 552 5 (pbk)

Contents

Acknowledgements

My special thanks to Bidwell Brook Special School, for letting me loose with the original idea and piloting the Profile, to Sue Stronge, speech & language therapist, for her invaluable help in getting this project off the ground, and to all my colleagues from the Speech and Language Therapy Department at South Devon Healthcare Trust for their encouragement and support.

I would also like to mention all my wonderful friends and their children, who have contributed without knowing it to the examples in this book — I've finally put the notebook away now, guys!

And to my parents, who started it all with a casual 'You could always become a speech & language therapist ...'

Figures

Figures

Introduction

The importance of involving the child's family and all those supporting the child in the planning and development of their communication programme is central to the idea behind the Communication Development Profile.

So many times reports are only accessible to those who share the same understanding, terminology and framework of development, and this can leave families and support workers uncertain about what is actually going on, and, at its worst, questioning the relevance of the targets and approach suggested.

The format of this Profile strives to provide a clear, shared framework of communication development which enables everyone involved to make informed contributions to a child's assessment and target setting, and to understand fully the resulting recommendations and programme. The Profile can either be photocopied and completed by hand or it can be done using the CD-ROM and stored electronically.

The Profile is not intended to be a stand-alone assessment but a way of explaining and making sense of observations and experiences of the child's communication. More detailed and formal assessments will be required in order to establish specific targets, and references are made throughout the Profile to other appropriate assessments and resources.

How to use the CD-ROM

Technical specifications

The interactive profile can be used on any Windows PC with the following minimum technical specifications:

* Operating System: Windows XP or Windows 2000

* Screen Resolution: 1024 x 768 or higher

* CD drive: x24 or higher

* The computer must not be set to disable .ini or .exe files

* The computer must allow the programme to write a folder and .txt files to the C:\ drive (My Documents folder)

* Microsoft Word must be installed

The programme will only run from the CD-ROM and cannot be installed on a computer.

How to complete the Profile

For a more detailed explanation of how to complete the profile see 'How to Complete the Profile' on page 5.

Creating a new profile

If you wish to start a new profile, follow these simple instructions:

* Place the CD-ROM in the CD drive and wait for the programme to start. It is always advisable to close down other programmes beforehand so that the CD-ROM can run at its optimum speed.

* From the **main menu** screen click on 'Create a new profile'. This will take you to a screen where you can fill in the child's name and the assessor's name. Simply click in the boxes you wish to type in. Today's date will automatically appear. You can change any of the type in the boxes in the usual way by selecting the text and either typing over it or deleting it.

* Next you will see a **profile menu** of all the questionnaires used to create the Profile. (You can also go to view the Profile screen, but at this stage it is blank.) Click on the questionnaire that you would like to start with.

* The nine questionnaires are divided into sections. Each section relates to a section on the Profile.

* Each item on the questionnaire has two empty boxes next to it: 'consistent level' and 'working within'. Click in any box and a tick will appear. To move a tick, click in the box you wish to move it to. To delete the tick altogether just click on it. Only when *all* the boxes for 'consistent level' in that section have been ticked will that section be recorded as 'consistent level' on the Profile. When some of the boxes for 'consistent level' have been ticked but not all, or if some of the 'working within' boxes have been ticked, the relevant section on the Profile will show 'working within'. If none of the boxes have been ticked in a particular section the profile section will be left blank.

* Each questionnaire has a comments box and information about where to find more information in the book. Click on the **information icon** ('*i*') for a brief description of what each item is assessing, and a page or chapter number where you can find more information in the book.

* A **comments box** at the base of each questionnaire page enables the user to describe the child's skills for that area. Click in the comments box and type. The box will scroll after a certain amount of text, so you can type as much as you want.

* The screen that follows the questionnaires enables you to summarise the child's overall profile or development levels and the communication phase that he is developing within. You can also use it for writing down any subsequent aims you might have for the child.

* When you have finished working on a questionnaire click on 'Profile' on the lower navigation bar to view the Profile. Otherwise you can return to the **profile menu**, print, or use the 'Next' and 'Back' buttons to work your way through as many of the questionnaires as you require.

Saving your profile

* The programme will save each profile that you make in a folder called 'CDP' that the programme will make for you, within the computer's 'My documents' folder. The programme will automatically name the file using the child's name, today's date and the name of the person completing the Profile.

- When you want to open a profile it will list all the files in that folder.

- There is also an option to save your files anywhere you wish, and change their name, if you already have your own filing system.

- There is a 'Save' icon on the Profile screen. If you try to leave the programme or return to the main menu without saving the profile, the 'Save' box will automatically appear.

Printing your profile

The Profile and the questionnaires can be printed out at any time to create a record of what has been achieved at each meeting with the child.

- To print a questionnaire that you have been working on go to that **questionnaire screen** and click on the 'Print' icon on the lower navigation menu.

- To print the Profile, go to the **profile screen** and do the same. To print both the Profile and all the questionnaires at the same time, go to the Profile screen and click on 'Print All'.

- To print blank copies of the Profile and questionnaires, choose 'Blank profile and questionnaires for printing' from the **main menu**, and then click on the item that you would like to print.

Opening a saved profile

Each time you want to amend a child's profile choose 'Open a saved profile' from the **main menu**.

- A box will appear, listing all the files that have been saved in the recommended folder. Click any of these to highlight a file then click on 'Open' if you want to look at a profile, or 'Delete' if you want to remove a profile.

- If you did not save your profile in the recommended folder, then you will have to use the 'Browse' button to locate it.

- Opening a profile will take you straight to the profile screen so that you can see how far you have got. Simply click on the area that you wish to work on that day, to take you to the relevant questionnaire. This will then be added to the Profile that you have already started, and a new file will be saved with that day's date so that a record of each session is maintained.

Key features of the *Communication Development Profile* on CD-ROM

1 Reassuring and easy to use, with help tips and information icons directing the assessor to where more information can be found in the book

2 Provides an at-a-glance visual representation of the child's communication skills

3 Easy to compare the relative stages of development across each area

4 A shareable resource that relates to both SLT and teaching assessments

5 An easily updateable format so that the child's progress can be charted over time

6 Case files are easily identifiable and searchable by using the 'save' facility with location and file-naming system

7 Completed profiles or blank copies can be printed and given to parents and teaching teams

8 The profile's design enables the SLT to give a visual representation of the child's development to parents and teaching teams

9 Enables parents and teaching teams to understand and be directly involved in the child's assessment and target setting

10 Helps to identify the most relevant form of support for the child's communication skills

11 A case study shows you how a typical profile of a child is built up using the nine questionnaires.

The Communication Development Profile
An overview

The key questions at the heart of many family and team discussions for a child with special needs are:

* Where is my/this child with respect to normal development?
* Where are things going wrong?
* What can I do to help?

How the Communication Development Profile works

The Communication Development Profile is designed to enable families, in particular, to be more directly involved in contributing to children's communication assessments and in planning their targets. The Profile helps speech & language therapists to explain their framework and decision-making to parents and teachers. It does so by breaking down the stages of communication development into small steps across the range of communication skills. Through evidence following assessment and/or from joint discussions with parents and teachers using the descriptions, the developmental stage for each communication skill is agreed. This information is then plotted onto a grid (see Profile 1) and provides the child's individual Communication Development Profile. An example of how the Communication Development Profile can be used, based on a real case history, is included on pages 113–123.

■ Area not relevant to the assessment

COMMUNICATION PHASES	COMMUNICATION STAGES	P-LEVEL	ATTENTION CONTROL	COMPREHENSION *What the child understands*	EXPRESSION *How the child communicates*	SOUND SYSTEM	USE OF COMMUNICATION *What and why the child communicates*	
EARLY COMMUNICATORS	INVOLUNTARY STAGE	P1(i/ii)				■		
	VOLUNTARY STAGE	P2(i)				■		
	'If I do … I get …'	P2(ii)	Fleeting attention			■		
	'If I do … You do …'	P3(i)						
DEVELOPING COMMUNICATORS	SITUATIONAL STAGE	P3(ii)		Situational understanding	Situational communication		Early intentions	
	FIRST WORDS *Single-word level*	P4	Own choice					First messages
	SIMPLE PHRASES *Two-word level*	P5	Adult control					
ESTABLISHED COMMUNICATORS	DESCRIBING PHRASES *Three-word level*	P6	Child control				Later intentions	
	GRAMMAR *Four-word level and above*	P7/P8	Two things at once					Conversational skills

Detailed descriptions of each stage of communication development

The Profile provides detailed descriptions of each stage of communication development, termed 'communication stages' starting from birth to the point at which a child understands and uses grammatical sentences.

* Involuntary stage
* Voluntary stage
* 'If I do ... I get ...' stage
* 'If I do ... You do ...' stage
* Situational stage

* First words
* Simple phrases
* Describing phrases
* Grammar and complex sentences

It identifies the underlying communicative competencies expected for each stage, and by matching them to the corresponding P-Level, enables speech & language therapists and teachers to use the same framework of communication development.

P-Levels are the performance descriptions set out in the DfEE/Qualification Curriculum Authority (QCA) Curriculum Guidelines (2005), which outline the eight levels of early learning and attainment leading up to Level 1 of the National Curriculum.

P-Levels can also be used in conjunction with the Foundation Curriculum (DfEE/QCA, 2003). However, it is important to realise that both the Foundation Curriculum and P-Levels have been written for different purposes and constructed in different ways. For children with significant special needs, P-Levels provide a more detailed and specific framework for assessment and planning.

For those establishments who do not use P-Levels the descriptive framework stands alone, and can still be used just as effectively to support joint discussions by referring to the speech & language terms only.

Assessment of the child across five key areas of communication

There are five main areas of communication, termed 'assessment areas', that speech & language therapists assess:

1 Attention Control (the child's ability to control and focus his own attention)
2 Comprehension (what the child understands)
3 Expression (how the child communicates)
4 Sound System (the development of the child's ability to produce and use sounds in words)
5 Use of Communication (what and why the child communicates)

This provides a wide range of information about the child's communication system, and enables the speech & language therapist to look at how each area is developing and how they interrelate and affect each other. Additional observations and assessments, such as the child's play skills and cognitive skills, help to further inform about how his communication development relates to his overall stage of development, which is also a very important consideration.

The communication phases

Communication development can be considered to move through three phases:

* Early Communicators
* Developing Communicators
* Established Communicators

These phases are derived from the development of a child's use of communication skills, as described by Gerard (1987) and by Anderson-Wood and Rae Smith (1997).

By establishing the communicative phase that a child is in, it is possible to identify the most developmentally appropriate style of intervention that will best support the child's communication skills at that point.

This has particular value in enabling the speech & language therapist to show, with evidence, when a child's needs will be best met either through the indirect management of their environment and everyday interactions, or through the direct approach of teaching language skills through specific activities. Doing this has considerable implications for the successful inclusion into educational placements such as nursery or school, of children whose communication skills fall within the Early or Developing Communicators phase. It is not enough just to provide a 'talking' environment; children need to be able to communicate meaningfully and equally, and to interact with the children and adults around them. This phase also emphasises that it is not just enhancing or changing the children's communication skills that makes the difference. In order for the child to make the most of the communication skills that they have, it is equally important that adults adapt their style of interaction and communication too, so that it best matches the child's developmental stage of communication.

How to Complete the Profile

Nine questionnaires are used to build up a child's profile. Most of the questionnaires are divided into sections, each section relating to one box on the Profile. Each item on the questionnaire has two empty boxes next to it to identify two skill levels:

* working within

* consistent level

The following shading has been used on the profile grid:

 Consistent level
The child uses the described skills on a daily basis, across different environments and situations, with minimal help or prompting.

 Working within
The child shows some development and independent use of the described skills but it is not consistent or established.

 Area not relevant to the assessment
The sound system is blacked out in the Early Communicators phase because although there is a development it is not an area that is relevant in planning at that stage.

The term 'working within' has been chosen very deliberately as this includes children who are maximising their skills rather than showing ongoing changes.

When the child has reached a consistent level on any of the items listed, simply tick the 'consistent level' box. If the child is still working towards that skill or if the child uses it inconsistently, then tick the 'working within' box. Only when all the boxes in that section have been ticked should that section be recorded as at a 'consistent level' on the Profile.

Please note that **only one level should be marked as 'working within' for each area of communication**.

Although some children may show splinter skills across the profile it is important to first identify the child's best, most consistent level for each area of communication (marked as the 'consistent level') and secondly to identify the next level above this where the child has not achieved all the skills (the 'working within' level).

Often when completing assessments and reports it is necessary to describe the level that the child is functioning at. However, few children fall neatly into any one level and simply stating that a child is at a particular stage neither gives enough information about what the child is achieving nor conveys their emerging skills. The Profile is designed to be a flexible indicator of the broad trends within the child's communication development and is *not a diagnostic assessment*.

Clearly, a clinical judgement does need to be made about which level the child is at, but the use of these levels enables the Profile to reflect both the child's underlying competencies, established through formal assessments, and their emerging skills, often reported by families and teaching staff or seen inconsistently in everyday situations.

The descriptions of each communication stage and assessment area in this book will support the discussions about why and how these results were gained and how they relate to the child in their everyday life.

Examples of typical scenarios and how the Profile helps to guide discussions

The most important thing is that the Profile is used to reflect the child's *communication development profile,* and in doing so helps everyone to make sense of what they are seeing and experiencing in their everyday interactions with the child.

It can be very reassuring for families to know that what they are worried about is, in fact, just a normal part of communication development, or that the area that they think is particularly delayed is actually at the point you would expect when compared with the other areas. Equally, it is very important that families and teaching staff understand exactly where the breakdown in communication is occurring – certainly problems in a child's use of communication skills are easily masked and misinterpreted as a breakdown in how the child is communicating, and the Profile is very useful in being able to show this distinction. For example:

Profiles 2 and 3 – using the Profile flexibly

Profile 2 (page 8) If a child is able to respond to a range of one-word-level commands but is only using a few words or signs independently with his expressive skills, by working from the single-word-level descriptions these can both be marked as 'working within' the 'first words' stage. The resulting Profile then reflects the expected pattern of development, that the child's understanding is slightly in advance of his expressive language skills but overall their development is balanced, in relation to each other.

Profile 3 (page 9) If, however, the speech & language therapist feels that there is enough evidence to suggest that the child's comprehension is showing some two-word level development, then the resulting profile would be used to show this imbalance, and priority may be given to supporting his expressive language development.

Profiles 4–8 (Chapter 1) and **Profiles 9–10** (Chapter 2) are examples (although neither exhaustive nor definitive) of typical situations which show how a visual representation of the different levels of communication can help to explain to parents and others what stage their child is at and to identify the key area needing support.

Profiles 4 and 5 – looking at how the child's expressive language and sound system relate to each other

A typical question might be:

I can't understand what my child is saying – why aren't you working on his sounds?

Profile 4 (page 10) indicates that the child's sound system development matches his language development, and reassures the parents that, although their child may still be difficult to understand and he cannot say all his sounds, this is exactly what you would expect at this stage of language development, and – most importantly – that working specifically on his speech sounds will not help to further develop his expressive language skills.

Profile 5 (page 11), however, highlights that the child's expected sound system development is behind his expressive language skills, and discussions may have to take place about how to best support him.

Profile 2 *Normal development, with all areas developing in line with each other*

COMMUNICATION PHASES	COMMUNICATION STAGES	P-LEVEL	ATTENTION CONTROL	COMPREHENSION *What the child understands*	EXPRESSION *How the child communicates*	SOUND SYSTEM	USE OF COMMUNICATION *What and why the child communicates*	
EARLY COMMUNICATORS	INVOLUNTARY STAGE	P1(i/ii)						
	VOLUNTARY STAGE	P2(i)						
	'If I do … I get …'	P2(ii)	Fleeting attention					
	'If I do … You do …'	P3(i)						
DEVELOPING COMMUNICATORS	SITUATIONAL STAGE	P3(ii)	Own choice	Situational understanding	Situational communication		Early intentions	First messages
	FIRST WORDS *Single-word level*	P4						
	SIMPLE PHRASES *Two-word level*	P5	Adult control					
ESTABLISHED COMMUNICATORS	DESCRIBING PHRASES *Three-word level*	P6	Child control				Later intentions	Conversational skills
	GRAMMAR *Four-word level and above*	P7/P8	Two things at once					

■ Area not relevant to the assessment   Consistent level   ▨ Working within

Profile 3 *The child's comprehension and expression development are unbalanced*

COMMUNICATION PHASES	COMMUNICATION STAGES	P-LEVEL	ATTENTION CONTROL	COMPREHENSION *What the child understands*	EXPRESSION *How the child communicates*	SOUND SYSTEM	USE OF COMMUNICATION *What and why the child communicates*	
EARLY COMMUNICATORS	INVOLUNTARY STAGE	P1(i/ii)				■		
	VOLUNTARY STAGE	P2(i)	Fleeting attention			■		
	'If I do … I get …'	P2(ii)				■		
	'If I do … You do …'	P3(i)				■		
DEVELOPING COMMUNICATORS	SITUATIONAL STAGE	P3(ii)	Own choice	Situational understanding	Situational communication		Early intentions	First messages
	FIRST WORDS *Single-word level*	P4						
	SIMPLE PHRASES *Two-word level*	P5	Adult control					
ESTABLISHED COMMUNICATORS	DESCRIBING PHRASES *Three-word level*	P6	Child control				Later intentions	Conversational skills
	GRAMMAR *Four-word level and above*	P7/P8	Two things at once					

■ Area not relevant to the assessment   ▒ Consistent level   ▨ Working within

Profile 4 *The child's sound system and expressive language developing in line with each other as expected*

COMMUNICATION PHASES	COMMUNICATION STAGES	P-LEVEL	ATTENTION CONTROL	COMPREHENSION *What the child understands*	EXPRESSION *How the child communicates*	SOUND SYSTEM	USE OF COMMUNICATION *What and why the child communicates*	
EARLY COMMUNICATORS	INVOLUNTARY STAGE	P1(i/ii)						
	VOLUNTARY STAGE	P2(i)						
	'If I do ... I get ...'	P2(ii)	Fleeting attention					
	'If I do ... You do ...'	P3(i)						
DEVELOPING COMMUNICATORS	SITUATIONAL STAGE	P3(ii)		Situational understanding	Situational communication			
	FIRST WORDS *Single-word level*	P4	Own choice				Early intentions	First messages
	SIMPLE PHRASES *Two-word level*	P5	Adult control					
ESTABLISHED COMMUNICATORS	DESCRIBING PHRASES *Three-word level*	P6	Child control					
	GRAMMAR *Four-word level and above*	P7/P8	Two things at once				Later intentions	Conversational skills

■ Area not relevant to the assessment   ▨ Consistent level   ▨ Working within

COMMUNICATION PHASES	COMMUNICATION STAGES	P-LEVEL	ATTENTION CONTROL	COMPREHENSION *What the child understands*	EXPRESSION *How the child communicates*	SOUND SYSTEM	USE OF COMMUNICATION *What and why the child communicates*
EARLY COMMUNICATORS	INVOLUNTARY STAGE	P1(i/ii)				■	
	VOLUNTARY STAGE	P2(i)				■	
	'If I do … I get …'	P2(ii)	Fleeting attention			■	
	'If I do … You do …'	P3(i)				■	
DEVELOPING COMMUNICATORS	SITUATIONAL STAGE	P3(ii)	Own choice	Situational understanding	Situational communication		First messages / Early intentions
	FIRST WORDS *Single-word level*	P4					
	SIMPLE PHRASES *Two-word level*	P5	Adult control				
ESTABLISHED COMMUNICATORS	DESCRIBING PHRASES *Three-word level*	P6	Child control				
	GRAMMAR *Four-word level and above*	P7/P8	Two things at once				Later intentions / Conversational skills

■ Area not relevant to the assessment   ▦ Consistent level   ▨ Working within

Profile 6 – the effect of the child's attention levels on his comprehension

Typical questions might be:

I find it really hard to work with this child. He ignores me or does his own thing a lot of the time but sometimes he amazes us with what he responds to.

Is it that he cannot understand what I am saying or is it his attention control that needs supporting?

Typically a child with difficulties in his attention control will show a pattern similar to **Profile 6** (page 13). His attention is fine when it is something of keen interest to him, he can respond to simple phrases some of the time and, as described, he even surprises people with his responses at other times, but then often seems to ignore other, simpler instructions. However, in contrast, he often uses long describing phrases appropriately and in context, and both the child's sound system and his use of language are also matched to this higher level.

This Profile gives a visual indicator that it is the child's attention control that is restricting his 'working' understanding, and that his inner language level is reflected when he is talking, particularly when he is in an informal situation and the listening demands on him are low. Discussions following this may well focus on how to support the child's attention control and what strategies to use in order to help him make it more effective, rather than on devising any targets for his understanding.

Profile 6 *A child with difficulties in attention control that affect his comprehension*

COMMUNICATION PHASES	COMMUNICATION STAGES	P-LEVEL	ATTENTION CONTROL	COMPREHENSION *What the child understands*	EXPRESSION *How the child communicates*	SOUND SYSTEM	USE OF COMMUNICATION *What and why the child communicates*
EARLY COMMUNICATORS	INVOLUNTARY STAGE	P1(i/ii)				▉	
	VOLUNTARY STAGE	P2(ii)	Fleeting attention			▉	
	'If I do ... I get ...'	P2(iii)				▉	
	'If I do ... You do ...'	P3(i)					First messages
DEVELOPING COMMUNICATORS	SITUATIONAL STAGE	P3(ii)		Situational understanding	Situational communication		
	FIRST WORDS *Single-word level*	P4	Own choice				Early intentions
	SIMPLE PHRASES *Two-word level*	P5	Adult control				
ESTABLISHED COMMUNICATORS	DESCRIBING PHRASES *Three-word level*	P6	Child control				Later intentions
	GRAMMAR *Four-word level and above*	P7/P8	Two things at once				Conversational skills

■ Area not relevant to the assessment   ▨ Consistent level   ▨ Working within

Profiles 7 and 8 – comparing the child's expressive language development with their use of these skills to communicate

> Typical concerns expressed by a parent might be:
>
> My son can say words and sentences – he is really good at using things he has heard, often from videos or his favourite sayings – but he does not seem to know how to use them to talk to me. I always seem to need to tell him what to say and get him to copy me. I want him to learn sentences so that he can ask for things he wants and tell me things without always being prompted.
>
> Can you get a communication aid for my child? I think it will help him to speak more.

In both these situations the core issue is the relationship between how the child communicates and his use of these skills to communicate.

Profile 7 (page 15) shows the child's expressive language skills in advance of his comprehension and attention skills and, most importantly, in advance of his use of communication skills.

In order to separate *how* the child communicates from his *use* of these skills, his expressive language is plotted on the profile so that it reflects his technical language skills – that is, the word combinations, typical sentence length and the maturity of grammatical information included in the sentences that the child is heard to use, even if they are learnt or copied phrases that are not used appropriately in context.

This is important, first, because it acknowledges the everyday experiences of the child's communication skills by his parents and teaching staff and, second, because the completed Profile then shows very clearly that:

* What the child is saying is more advanced than what he understands and responds to. As a result, it can be better explained that the child in this example probably does not understand the individual words that he is saying, and is therefore unlikely to be able to use these same words in a variety of new or different sentences. In fact, his comprehension level (working within simple phrases) is probably more indicative of his overall baseline language levels.

* And, most significantly, the Profile also indicates that what the child is saying is in advance of his ability to use his sentences to communicate. Again, this helps to make sense of why the child is not communicating spontaneously with the language he has. It is not the child's spoken language skills that need further support, but his ability to use the language skills that he has already in order to communicate a range

Profile 7 *Expressive language skills in advance of use of communication skills*

COMMUNICATION PHASES	COMMUNICATION STAGES	P-LEVEL	ATTENTION CONTROL	COMPREHENSION *What the child understands*	EXPRESSION *How the child communicates*	SOUND SYSTEM	USE OF COMMUNICATION *What and why the child communicates*
EARLY COMMUNICATORS	INVOLUNTARY STAGE	P1(i/ii)					
	VOLUNTARY STAGE	P2(i)	Fleeting attention				
	'If I do … I get …'	P2(ii)					
	'If I do … You do …'	P3(i)					
DEVELOPING COMMUNICATORS	SITUATIONAL STAGE	P3(ii)		Situational understanding	Situational communication		
	FIRST WORDS *Single-word level*	P4	Own choice				Early intentions
	SIMPLE PHRASES *Two-word level*	P5	Adult control				
ESTABLISHED COMMUNICATORS	DESCRIBING PHRASES *Three-word level*	P6	Child control				First messages
	GRAMMAR *Four-word level and above*	P7/P8	Two things at once				Later intentions / Conversational skills

■ Area not relevant to the assessment   ▨ Consistent level   ▨ Working within

of messages and early intentions, and to be able to do so independently, without prompts. Of course, whether the child then chooses to communicate about these things is a different issue!

It is important to point out that things are never simple when it comes to unpicking a child's communication skills and trying to identify the point of breakdown. Many children will use learnt chunks of language quite appropriately – in fact they seem to need to learn their language skills in this 'cut and paste' way. However, what differentiates these children from the example above is that their expressive language skills and use of communication skills are generally better balanced.

Another scenario occurs when both the child's comprehension and expression are at the higher level, in advance of their *use of communication*. Again, this highlights that this area needs support rather than the child's language skills (see Profile 12, page 26).

Profile 8 (page 17) Communication aids are great for supporting a child whose use of communication is in advance of his expressive language skills (how the child communicates) and sound system. Usually these are children who have a real drive and motivation to communicate, and manage to get their messages across using whatever skills they have, but, for whatever reason, have limited physical skills.

Providing a more reliable way for these children to communicate can be the most important thing that we do, as it enhances their success as communicators and supports their ongoing development in the use of communication far more effectively and usefully than trying to improve their physical abilities.

It is important to remember that communication aids do not primarily support the development of, or provide the motivation for, a child to want to communicate (see Chapter 8), and if his use of communication skills are matched to, or in advance of, his expressive language skills then it is unlikely that providing a communication aid will help.

Finally, please remember, as mentioned at the beginning of this section, that the Profiles and discussions above are neither exhaustive nor definitive. They merely demonstrate the way that the Communication Development Profile can be used to support discussions and the broad trends that can be seen.

Profile 8 *Use of communication skills in advance of the child's expressive language skills*

COMMUNICATION PHASES	COMMUNICATION STAGES	P-LEVEL	ATTENTION CONTROL	COMPREHENSION *What the child understands*	EXPRESSION *How the child communicates*	SOUND SYSTEM	USE OF COMMUNICATION *What and why the child communicates*	
EARLY COMMUNICATORS	INVOLUNTARY STAGE	P1(i/ii)				■		
	VOLUNTARY STAGE	P2(i)	Fleeting attention			■		
	'If I do … I get …'	P2(ii)				■		
	'If I do … You do …'	P3(i)				■		
DEVELOPING COMMUNICATORS	SITUATIONAL STAGE	P3(ii)		Situational understanding	Situational communication			
	FIRST WORDS *Single-word level*	P4	Own choice				Early intentions	First messages
	SIMPLE PHRASES *Two-word level*	P5	Adult control					
ESTABLISHED COMMUNICATORS	DESCRIBING PHRASES *Three-word level*	P6	Child control				Later intentions	Conversational skills
	GRAMMAR *Four-word level and above*	P7/P8	Two things at once					

■ Area not relevant to the assessment ▨ Consistent level ▦ Working within

The Communication Phases & Intervention

The one certainty about intervention is that it is always changing according to research, trends and current evidence.

The Communication Development Profile helps to identify the style of speech & language therapy that best matches the child's communication development stage and, most importantly, his stage of pragmatic development (use of communication skills): see Anderson-Wood and Rae Smith (1997).

The following information outlines each of the communication phases, and discusses how they can be used to inform and shape the way we provide speech & language therapy intervention and everyday support to children with communication difficulties.

Phase 1: Early Communicators

Children are learning how to be communicators, so that they can influence the world around them and, crucially, so that they can interact with and influence other people. During this phase children use a whole range of behaviours, from crying, facial movements and expressions to reaching, looking and making noises, and they progress from using their behaviours in response to things going on around them, to using them in a planned and deliberate manner in order to achieve a specific goal.

Broadly, this phase covers:

* INVOLUNTARY REFLEXES AND REACTIONS	**P1(i) and P1(ii)**
* VOLUNTARY REACTIONS	**P2(i)**
* 'IF I DO …I GET …': PURPOSEFUL ACTIONS	**P2(ii)**
* 'IF I DO … YOU DO …': EARLY THREE-WAY COMMUNICATION	**P3(i)**

Intervention to support children in their interactions with other people, and for them to be able to make their needs, choices and preferences known, depends entirely upon the people in the child's environment. For example, a very good framework for creating a responsive environment comes from Jean Ware (1996), who defines it as one in which children:

* Get responses to their actions
* Have the opportunity to give responses
* Have an opportunity to take the lead in interactions

Good practice includes the creation of a 'Personal Communication Passport' (Millar & Aitken, 2003) enabling everyone to share the way that the child reacts and behaves, leading to more consistent and sensitive responses by the adults, and, ultimately, that the child is seen to be, and treated as, a communicator.

Phase 2: Developing Communicators

Within this phase children are gaining language-based skills, they are beginning to use sounds and words to mean things and can understand and respond to a growing range of words; however, they are developing these skills without realising it, through the process of closely matched adult–child interactions rather than being specifically taught. For example, the child points at the car and says 'dah'; the adult looks around and responds with 'yes, Mummy's car', reinforcing the child's message and adding more words; the child may even then copy what he has heard, 'mu dah', further reinforcing his learning. This phase of communication development can therefore be considered as a largely unconscious learning process for both children and adults.

Broadly it includes the development of:
* SITUATIONAL STAGE   *Established three-way communication*   **P3(ii)**
* FIRST WORDS   *Single-word level*   **P4**
* SIMPLE PHRASES   *Two-word level*   **P5**

In terms of intervention, given that for the majority of this phase the child finds taking directions for tasks very hard and gives his best attention to things that are highly interesting and self-motivating, direct teaching of language skills is clearly not going to achieve the optimum learning environment. After all, if you are involved in an ongoing battle to gain and maintain a child's attention, he will have little attention left to take notice of the content of your session, however appropriate it seemed on paper! Intervention to support children's use and development of their communication skills therefore needs to focus on creating these naturalistic and highly responsive interactions, which are described by Tannock et al (1992) as the adult's language and style of communicating being equally matched, and responsive to, the children's focus of attention.

In order to achieve balanced interaction, therefore, it is important that adults adapt their style to work within a child's best attention levels by:
* Following the child's lead, and talking about what the child is looking at and doing
* Adding to and expanding on what the child has said
* Using play-based activities that are interesting and motivating to the child
* Making the most of real, everyday situations and opportunities to communicate

Useful sources of information to support this include the Hanen Centre, 'I CAN' Course, PCI and Child (2004).

Phase 3: Established Communicators

Within this phase children are gaining increasingly sophisticated language-based skills; they are now able to understand and respond to a much wider range of words, including those that describe concepts such as colour, position and timescale; and they are also beginning to use these words in longer and more complex sentences.

Most significantly, because children now understand what language is all about and how it works (sometimes described as 'meta-linguistic skills') they are able to make direct changes to their language skills, through adding new words or structures and amending others. For example, the child uses the word 'up' instead of 'on' and, by the adult correcting him, he gradually replaces it. The whole language-learning process has become deliberate and conscious, and children developing within this stage can learn language through language.

This phase, therefore, includes the development of:

* DESCRIBING PHRASES   *Three-word level*   **P6**
* GRAMMAR AND COMPLEX SENTENCES *Four-word level and above*   **P7 and P8**

Intervention which aims to change a child's speech or language skills can now take place effectively through direct intervention with the child; the adult involvement is in building the child's understanding of the underlying language and concepts and in correcting and modifying their spoken language. This is seen as the more traditional or table top form of speech & language therapy.

Of course, language development does not stop here; there is a range of higher language skills which develop after this point, and these are covered more fully in other speech and language assessments, and from Level 1 of the National Curriculum.

> **Why isn't my child receiving direct speech & language therapy?**
> **The value in using these phases in planning and explaining intervention.**

The child's communication phase is established in two ways: it is either taken from the phase in which the child's overall 'working within' level falls, or, if his skills are plotted across two phases, the one in which his 'working within' level for his use of communication skills falls.

In their book, Andersen-Wood and Rae Smith (1997) point out that it is the level of a child's use of communication skills (pragmatic skills) that should inform the most developmentally appropriate style of intervention: 'It is our impression that many of the problems encountered in treating pragmatic difficulties can be attributed to working at too high a developmental level for the individual client.' I would add that, from my experience, this holds true for working on any aspect of communication skills for a child with special needs. If the style of intervention is aimed at direct teaching activities when the child is still developing his skills within the Developing Communicators phase, and therefore learning best through a closely matched interaction, then it is likely that not only will the approach be ineffective but, worse still, the people around the child may feel he is not suitable for 'therapy' or 'this school or that school'. Simply matching the best style of intervention to the child's communication phase, and in particular focussing on the development of the child's use of communication skills, rather than his language skills, helps to overcome a lot of these difficulties.

Of course, this is challenging when a child is included within a mainstream school and his best style of intervention is a play-based, interactive one, whilst everyone else is working with a table top style. However, it is even more important then that these phases are used. They help to inform the parents and teaching team about the child's needs and to support the way that they work with the child; they also help to provide people with realistic expectations both for the child and for themselves, and they help to explain the speech & language therapist's role in supporting them. Most importantly, where this framework is used, it helps to put the child and his needs at the centre of it all.

Examples of profiles showing the communication phase the child is 'working within'

Profile 9 (page 23) The child is working within the Early Communicators phase and needs a highly sensitive and responsive communication environment.

Profile 10 (page 24) The child is working within the Developing Communicators phase and will learn best from a closely matched adult–child interaction.

Profile 11 (page 25) The child is working within the Established Communicators phase and can therefore learn language through language, and cope with direct teaching techniques and table top activities.

Profile 12 (page 26) The child's use of communication skills is still developing within the Developing Communicators phase; therefore intervention is best provided through indirect targets to match and support this level of development, rather than direct targets.

Profile 9 *The child is working within the Early Communicators phase and needs a highly sensitive and responsive communication environment.*

COMMUNICATION PHASES	COMMUNICATION STAGES	P-LEVEL	ATTENTION CONTROL	COMPREHENSION *What the child understands*	EXPRESSION *How the child communicates*	SOUND SYSTEM	USE OF COMMUNICATION *What and why the child communicates*	
EARLY COMMUNICATORS	INVOLUNTARY STAGE	P1(i/ii)						
	VOLUNTARY STAGE	P2(i)						
	'If I do … I get …'	P2(ii)	Fleeting attention					
	'If I do … You do …'	P3(i)						
DEVELOPING COMMUNICATORS	SITUATIONAL STAGE	P3(ii)		Situational understanding	Situational communication		Early intentions	First messages
	FIRST WORDS *Single-word level*	P4	Own choice					
	SIMPLE PHRASES *Two-word level*	P5	Adult control					
ESTABLISHED COMMUNICATORS	DESCRIBING PHRASES *Three-word level*	P6	Child control				Later intentions	Conversational skills
	GRAMMAR *Four-word level and above*	P7/P8	Two things at once					

■ Area not relevant to the assessment   Consistent level   ▨ Working within

COMMUNICATION PHASES	COMMUNICATION STAGES	P-LEVEL	ATTENTION CONTROL	COMPREHENSION *What the child understands*	EXPRESSION *How the child communicates*	SOUND SYSTEM	USE OF COMMUNICATION *What and why the child communicates*	
EARLY COMMUNICATORS	INVOLUNTARY STAGE	P1(i/ii)						
	VOLUNTARY STAGE	P2(i)						
	'If I do … I get …'	P2(ii)	Fleeting attention					
	'If I do … You do …'	P3(i)						
DEVELOPING COMMUNICATORS	SITUATIONAL STAGE	P3(ii)		Situational understanding	Situational communication			
	FIRST WORDS *Single-word level*	P4	Own choice				Early intentions	First messages
	SIMPLE PHRASES *Two-word level*	P5	Adult control					
ESTABLISHED COMMUNICATORS	DESCRIBING PHRASES *Three-word level*	P6	Child control				Later intentions	Conversational skills
	GRAMMAR *Four-word level and above*	P7/P8	Two things at once					

■ Area not relevant to the assessment   ▢ Consistent level   ▨ Working within

Profile 11   *The child is working within the Established Communicators phase and can therefore learn language through language, and cope with direct teaching techniques and table top activities.*

COMMUNICATION PHASES	COMMUNICATION STAGES	P-LEVEL	ATTENTION CONTROL	COMPREHENSION *What the child understands*	EXPRESSION *How the child communicates*	SOUND SYSTEM	USE OF COMMUNICATION *What and why the child communicates*	
EARLY COMMUNICATORS	INVOLUNTARY STAGE	P1(i/ii)						
	VOLUNTARY STAGE	P2(i)	Fleeting attention					
	"If I do … I get … "	P2(ii)						
	"If I do … You do … "	P3(i)						
DEVELOPING COMMUNICATORS	SITUATIONAL STAGE	P3(ii)		Situational understanding	Situational communication			
	FIRST WORDS *Single-word level*	P4	Own choice				Early intentions	First messages
	SIMPLE PHRASES *Two-word level*	P5	Adult control					
ESTABLISHED COMMUNICATORS	DESCRIBING PHRASES *Three-word level*	P6	Child control				Later intentions	Conversational skills
	GRAMMAR *Four-word level and above*	P7/P8	Two things at once					

■ **Area not relevant to the assessment**   ▨ **Consistent level**   ▨ **Working within**

Profile 12 *The child's use of communication skills is still developing within the Developing Communicators phase; therefore intervention is best provided through indirect targets to match and support this level of development, rather than direct targets.*

COMMUNICATION PHASES	COMMUNICATION STAGES	P-LEVEL	ATTENTION CONTROL	COMPREHENSION *What the child understands*	EXPRESSION *How the child communicates*	SOUND SYSTEM	USE OF COMMUNICATION *What and why the child communicates*	
EARLY COMMUNICATORS	INVOLUNTARY STAGE	P1(i/ii)						
	VOLUNTARY STAGE	P2(i)	Fleeting attention					
	'If I do ... I get ...'	P2(ii)						
	'If I do ... You do ...'	P3(i)						
DEVELOPING COMMUNICATORS	SITUATIONAL STAGE	P3(ii)	Own choice	Situational understanding	Situational communication		Early intentions	First messages
	FIRST WORDS *Single-word level*	P4						
	SIMPLE PHRASES *Two-word level*	P5	Adult control					
ESTABLISHED COMMUNICATORS	DESCRIBING PHRASES *Three-word level*	P6	Child control				Later intentions	Conversational skills
	GRAMMAR *Four-word level and above*	P7/P8	Two things at once					

■ Area not relevant to the assessment   ▨ Consistent level   ▨ Working within

Attention Control

A child's ability to listen, and to attend to what is happening and to what is being said, is a fundamental part of being able to respond appropriately to both verbal and non-verbal information. There are an enormous number of reasons why a child will find developing these skills difficult; however, the following structure, based on the well-known model by Cooper et al (1978), is very useful in identifying the child's developmental stage for attention control. By comparing this with the child's stage of development for his understanding and expression, it helps to indicate whether the child has a specific difficulty in this area or whether the child's level of attention is what you would expect for his overall stage of development.

Early Communicators

Fleeting attention

P-Levels ✻ **P1(i)–P3(i)**

During this phase a child cannot control his own focus of attention, so it moves rapidly from one thing to another, usually to whatever is the most dominant or interesting thing happening around him. The child could be described as highly distractible.

Gaining and maintaining a child's attention is best done through sharing an interest in what he is doing or looking at, responding to his noises and actions, starting games that you know he likes and adapting to his frequent change in focus.

Developing Communicators

Own choice

P-Levels ✻ **P3(ii) and P4**

The child is now able to focus and maintain his attention on an activity that is highly interesting or motivating, but he has his own idea of what he wants to do and is unlikely to be interested in your choice of activity, or in playing a game by your rules.

For some children any attempt to join in an activity or give them suggestions of what to do next will result in their ignoring you and sticking to their own agenda. Other children will be completely distracted by another person joining in and unable to maintain their focus of attention and, as a result, are likely to wander off and find something else to play with.

Routledge P
Taylor & Francis Group
ROUTLEDGE

Within this stage a child's best attention is gained and maintained through joining in with an activity or setting up one that interests and motivates him. It is important that the adult is totally undemanding in their style, following the child's lead and showing interest in his game rather than telling him what to do; this may include giving a simple running commentary on what he is doing, responding to the child's noises and actions, and copying his play. The key thing is that asking questions and giving instructions should be kept to an absolute minimum.

Adult control *single-channelled*

P-Level   P5

The child can now have his attention focussed by an adult, and can take directions from the adult, but he can only pay his full looking and listening attention to one thing at a time (single-channelled attention); he cannot listen and do at the same time. This makes it difficult for a child to shift his attention between what he is doing to what is being said, and he is therefore reliant on the adult gaining and maintaining his attention before giving instructions and throughout directed activities (adult control).

A child's best attention is gained and maintained by ensuring that the child is giving you his full looking and listening attention before you give an instruction or information. This will mean interrupting the activity that the child is currently involved in (playing, watching television, the task you are doing with him) and making sure he is not fiddling or distracted whilst he is listening. In other words, instructions are best given 'outside' the task itself.

Other tips include starting an instruction with the child's name, so that he is aware that you are speaking to him right from the beginning, and making sure that you speak to him from in front and as much as possible at his level – talking from behind, above, across the room or even by his side can reduce a child's ability to be able to focus on what you are saying.

Established Communicators
Child control *single-channelled*

P-Level   P6

The child still needs to give his full looking and listening attention to one thing at a time (so is still single-channelled) but his attention is much more flexible and under his own control, so he can now shift his own focus of attention between the activity and what is being said. Adults may still need to ensure they have gained the child's attention before they speak, particularly in busy and distracting situations, but they will need fewer strategies to do so.

Routledge
Taylor & Francis Group
ROUTLEDGE

The child's best attention is gained and maintained by following strategies similar to those outlined above under 'adult control', but as the child becomes better at controlling and shifting his own attention, these will be needed less frequently.

Two things at once *two-channelled*

Short periods

P-Level · P7

The child can now pay attention to, and concentrate on, two things at once: he can listen to an adult giving him instructions or information about the task without stopping what he is doing. He is able to take directions 'within' the task.

Integrated and sustained

P-Level · P8

The child can maintain two-channelled attention for long periods, and for unrelated topics; he can watch television whilst talking about school.

The child is now able to control and maintain his own focus of attention independently from what is going on around him, and these dual attention skills mean he can now learn effectively in a group situation because he is no longer switching off when it is someone else's turn. This is the level of attention that is needed to be able to learn within a busy and distracting environment and during large group work.

> **KEY POINT**
> A child's attention levels will fluctuate for a number of reasons – it is helpful to agree the overall, most consistent level of attention control and then to note his best and worst situations, so that the parents and carers will have a balanced profile.

Attention Control – Overview of Developmental Stages

Early Communicators	P-LEVEL
✱ FLEETING ATTENTION	**P1(i)–P3(i)**
Developing Communicators	
✱ OWN CHOICE	**P3(ii) and P4**
✱ ADULT CONTROL (SINGLE-CHANNELLED)	**P5**
Established Communicators	
✱ CHILD CONTROL (SINGLE-CHANNELLED)	**P6**
✱ TWO THINGS AT ONCE (TWO-CHANNELLED)	
– SHORT PERIODS	**P7**
– INTEGRATED AND SUSTAINED	**P8**

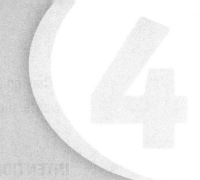

The Development of Intentional Communication

This page may be photocopied for instructional use only. *The Communication Development Profile* © Charlotte Child 2006

From birth, children react to things going on inside them and around them. Gradually these reactions and changes in behaviour become planned and controlled by the child. Eventually the child begins to deliberately aim his behaviour at the adult in order to give a message. In the early stage, it is rather hit and miss, but by the established stage the adult is in no doubt that the child is communicating a message, and we describe the child as being an 'intentional communicator'. Using the following framework based on work by Coupe O'Kane and Goldbart (1998) enables us to consider all children to be communicators, however subtle their behaviour, and to provide the most responsive interaction environment that we can.

Pre-intentional Stages of Communication Development

1. Involuntary reactions and reflexes

| P-Levels | P1(i) and P1(ii) |

In the early stages after birth, the child has a small range of involuntary movements and behaviours which are not under his deliberate control and are triggered as reactions to the child's body sensations and to very strong external events.

2. Voluntary reactions

| P-Level | P2(i) |

Gradually the child is able to make and control a wider range of movements which, owing to his greater awareness and interest in things going on externally to himself, he uses as reactions to people, events and objects.

3. 'If I do ... I get ...' purposeful actions

| P-Level | P2(ii) |

In this stage of communicative development the child begins to explore and create changes in his immediate environment through movements and actions which are becoming planned and purposeful. The child is learning that 'if he does this ... then that happens'. This can therefore be called 'If I do ... I get ...' because it describes the change to children being active in trying to do things for themselves and learning what they need to do in order to get what they want.

This 'having a go' can be described as 'goal-directed behaviour', as the child knows what he wants and goes for it, or more simply as 'I know what I want' behaviour.

INTENTIONAL BEHAVIOUR – 'I know what I want'

A child's behaviour can be described as goal-directed or intentional when the following five features can be observed:

1 The child has a goal in mind: for example, he wants the noisy toy to work/wants a biscuit from the cupboard

2 The child has a go at achieving his goal, that is, by pulling the string/trying to open the cupboard door

3 The child maintains and persists with this behaviour until it is successful, that is, he keeps pulling the string until it works/pulling the door until it opens

4 The child stops his actions once he has achieved his goal; that is, he sits and watches the noisy toy working/gets and eats the biscuit.

5 If the child does not achieve his goal he modifies his approach and continues; that is, he tries to find another way of making it work – for example he may drop or throw the toy/climb up onto the cupboard or pull even harder at the door and scream angrily at it!

O'Kane & Goldbart (1998)

By its very nature, then, children who are not able to physically 'have a go' and manipulate their environment will need lots of sensitive interactions and opportunities to enable them to experience control in their lives and to learn goal-directed behaviour through other means.

This page may be photocopied for instructional use only. *The Communication Development Profile* © Charlotte Child 2006

Routledge
Taylor & Francis Group
ROUTLEDGE

Intentional Stages of Communication Development

The significant change is in the child's changing his behaviour from doing things for himself to using his behaviour to get people to do things for him, ie change from 'I know what I want', intentional behaviour to 'I'm telling you what I want', intentional communicative behaviour. It can also be described as 'If I do … You do …'

However, it is easier said than done, and the child's first attempts are generally dodgy, with the child seeming unclear whose attention he is trying to gain and why! It is therefore useful to describe this development at two levels:

4. 'If I do … You do …' purposeful communication strategies

P-Level   P3(i)

This can be described as 'early three-way communication'. The child uses a range of behaviours to try to involve the adult and communicate a message, but he tends to direct these at either the adult or the object but does not manage to coordinate both at once. It is an early stage of intentional communication.

5. 'And I won't give up!' situational communication

P-Level   P3(ii)

This can be described as 'established three-way communication'. The child has a range of more recognisable communicative behaviours which he uses to gain the adult's attention and then direct it to what he wants them to do or to look at, and will persist until he has achieved his goal, hence the phrase 'And I won't give up!' It is within this stage that a child generally develops fully intentional communicative behaviour.

Routledge
Taylor & Francis Group
ROUTLEDGE

INTENTIONAL COMMUNICATIVE BEHAVIOUR – 'I'm telling you what I want'

A child's communicative behaviour can be considered to be fully intentional when the following four features can be observed:

1 The use of attention-seeking behaviour to get an adult involved, for example screaming and shouting/looking at the adult whilst vocalising

2 Persistence and repetition of behaviours until the child gets what he wants, for example more screaming and shouting with (depending on the level of communication) some other behaviour such as reaching or looking towards what the child is after/continuing to look at the adult and vocalising

3 Changing tactics if he is not successful, for example a full-blown tantrum/ making the vocalisations louder and more protesting

4 Satisfaction on achieving his goal, that is, peace at last as the adult has finally found out what the child wanted

Stephenson & Linfoot (1996)

In order for children to have the best opportunity to make this transition, it underlines the importance of everyone seeing the child as being communicative, and the sensitive and consistent interpretation of his behaviours at this point, particularly if his responses are slow, unpredictable or hard to interpret (Ware, 1996).

Other children will learn how to communicate through direct actions on people and things, ie will be able to use purposeful communication strategies, but find the transition into the distance and true signalling communication in the next stage – situational communication – very difficult.

Communication – Overview of Developmental Stages

Pre-intentional stages	P-LEVEL
* INVOLUNTARY REACTIONS AND REFLEXES	**P1(i) and P1(ii)**
* VOLUNTARY REACTIONS	**P2(i)**
* 'IF I DO … I GET …': PURPOSEFUL ACTIONS	**P2(ii)**
Intentional stages	
* 'IF I DO … YOU DO …': PURPOSEFUL COMMUNICATION STRATEGIES (EARLY THREE-WAY COMMUNICATION)	**P3(i)**
* 'AND I WON'T GIVE UP!': SITUATIONAL COMMUNICATION (ESTABLISHED THREE-WAY COMMUNICATION)	**P3(ii)**

Comprehension
What the child understands

In the Early Communicators phase, the child's comprehension is observed as the things that he responds to. Initially the child responds to things happening to and within himself; this gradually changes to include responses to external things and events; then the child learns to interpret what an adult means by their actions: and finally, in the Developing Communicators phase, the child begins to understand and respond to words.

Being able to understand what has been said involves the development of a number of different skills:

* The range of words that the child can understand (naming, action, describing)
* The number of words that the child can respond to in a sentence
* The amount of grammatical information that he can understand
* The child's ability to cope with complex sentences, working out the meaning irrespective of how the words are organised or sequenced
* The child's ability to understand the meanings conveyed through non-verbal communication, such as tone of voice and facial expression, which can override the literal meaning of the words, as with sarcasm and moods

The development of these skills is, to a great extent, reliant on the child's ability to:

* Listen and control his focus of attention (attention control)
* Remember what has been said long enough to work out the meaning, and respond (auditory memory)
* Understand the world around him (cognitive skills)

A child's ability to understand what has been said to him can break down within any one, or a combination of, these areas and can cause significant difficulties.

How do you work out the child's 'word level' for his understanding of spoken language (comprehension)?

> The word level for the child's understanding of spoken language equals the number of 'key information words' that the child has understood from an instruction.

Routledge
Taylor & Francis Group
ROUTLEDGE

What is a 'Key Information Word'?

A 'key information word' is a term used to describe a word that the child *has* to know and respond to in order to get the instruction right. One way of determining a child's comprehension level is by finding out the number of key information words that the child is consistently able to respond to. Children may appear to respond to all the words that you say, but it is important to consider how much was obvious from the situation and how much could only be understood from the words.

As a general rule, for a word to be a key information word there need to be other choices available for the child to think about so that you can be sure that the child has responded correctly to the word, rather than by chance, for example, 'Give the cup to Grandma'.

If the child is holding the cup and you point him in the direction of Grandma, he has not had to think much about the words that you said. When there are no other options and the meaning is obvious from the situation or from what the adult is doing, it does not count. The child could just be responding to the adult's actions rather than the words. Even words like 'give' and 'put' are generally redundant because the child can usually guess from the situation what you expect him to do with the items — and if he does not, the adult prompts him by pointing, reaching or helping.

However, if there were a number of different items on the table and the child, without any help, picked up the cup rather than the spoon, and gave it to Grandma rather than to Grandpa, you could say that the child had to think about and make choices between the options for 'cup' and 'Grandma'.

Therefore, in this situation, where there are alternative choices for the words *cup* and *Grandma*, these are considered the *key information words* for that instruction.

Alternative terms used include '*information-carrying words*' and '*key words*'.

In real life this can be very difficult to work out — therefore more formal assessments are very important because by setting up controlled situations using toys, objects or pictures, and being careful to ensure that there is no help from the situation or the people around the child, it is clear what the language load is and what the available choices are.

Even then it is still not straightforward — children who do not have directable attention will not be able to respond to the instructions, irrespective of whether or not they understood them, and this prevents an accurate assessment of what they may be able to understand. In addition, the situation, toys and other factors play a large part in the child's performance, which is why the combined observations of everyone help to pull the whole picture together; it is important to consider the child's overall pattern of responses to a range of vocabulary (naming, action and describing words) and grammar, and not just the number of key words that the child responds to.

Routledge P Taylor & Francis Group. This page may be photocopied for instructional use only. *The Communication Development Profile* © Charlotte Child 2006

Comprehension – Overview of Developmental Stages

Early Communicators		P-LEVEL
* INVOLUNTARY REACTIONS AND REFLEXES		**P1(i) and P1(ii)**
* VOLUNTARY REACTIONS		**P2(i)**
* 'IF I DO … I GET …'		**P2(ii)**
* 'IF I DO … YOU DO …'		**P3(i)**
Developing Communicators		
* SITUATIONAL UNDERSTANDING		**P3(ii)**
* UNDERSTANDING FIRST WORDS	*Single-word level*	**P4**
* UNDERSTANDING SIMPLE PHRASES	*Two-word level*	**P5**
Established Communicators		
* UNDERSTANDING DESCRIBING PHRASES	*Three-word level*	**P6**
* UNDERSTANDING GRAMMAR AND COMPLEX SENTENCES		**P7 and P8**
	Four-word level and above	

Each of these stages is explained in detail on pages 40–58.

Routledge
Taylor & Francis Group
ROUTLEDGE

Early Communicators

The child uses a small range of movements and behaviours as **reactions to**:

* Something happening to himself: **P-Level P1(i)**
  Hunger
  Thirst
  Discomfort
  Pain

* Something happening around him: **P-Level P1(ii)**
  A loud noise
  A sudden movement
  Strong light changes

Routledge
Taylor & Francis Group
ROUTLEDGE

The child has developed a greater awareness and interest in things going on externally to himself and can now use his movements and behaviours as **reactions to**:

* Familiar people (eg increasing his arm and leg movements while an adult gives him attention)
* Toys or objects (eg by holding or looking at)
* Events (eg to food and drink approaching – by opening his mouth in anticipation)

Anticipation and turn-taking begins to develop within predictable, everyday, routine activities and repetitive games. From these the child learns to recognise what is happening at that moment, as it is happening. For example, he recognises that it is bathtime because he is being washed in the bath.

The child is now developing a much better understanding of the real world around him, what goes on in it and what he can expect to happen within his daily routines, which leads to more **purposeful responses** in relation to the following:

Events

The child's understanding of events in his daily routine means he can now anticipate what is about to happen next. For example:

∗ The child knows it is bathtime when he is in the bathroom being undressed and can hear his bath running.
∗ The child knows it is time for juice when he sees it being prepared.
∗ The child knows that he is going out as his shoes are picked up and put on.

In addition, if what the child is anticipating does not happen, or there is a change to the routine that he does not want or does not like, he will respond to this using a range of (generally loud) protesting behaviours, for example, if his drink does not arrive quickly enough (by his standards), or if the adult disappears out of sight holding his cup instead of bringing it straight to him.

Events that the child likes or is interested in will be responded to by quiet satisfaction and exploration. (You should already be getting the idea that children learn to communicate first about what they do *not* want!)

Objects

The ability to use purposeful actions on the environment and the things in it lead to the child's learning to respond more specifically to an object. For example, the child learns to shake a shaky thing, push a pushing thing, chew a chewy thing and visually explore small things in great detail, which gradually replaces the 'chew it and chuck it all' approach.

People

The child will show some reactions to:

∗ Changes in adults' intonation and voice quality – particularly to angry and to happy voices
∗ Changes in adults' facial expressions – particularly to cross looks and to smiles
∗ Some actions – such as responding to adults' holding out their arms to offer a hug

At this point the child will readily respond to 'people games', that is, games which focus entirely on joint play between the adult and child without an object being a main part of it, for example, peek-a-boo, tickling games ('This Little Piggy', 'Round and Round the Garden') and physical action games ('Down at the Bottom of the Deep Blue Sea').

'If I do ... You do ...'
purposeful communication strategies

The child is beginning to understand and respond to the **adult's actions**, and in this way begins to cooperate and take an active part in everyday routines. For example, the child will respond to:

* An object held out for him by an adult (by taking it)
* A hand that is held out for him (by taking it)
* Where the adult is pointing (by looking in the same direction)*
* To 'No' with intonation (by pausing in what he is doing)
* He will also begin to respond to gestures for 'Give me', 'Come here' and 'Sit down', as long as he is also being directly helped to do it
* In addition, the child starts to actively watch an adult's face and gestures for clues

However, the child will need lots of direct help and encouragement to do so; for example, the adult will typically:

* Call the child's name, whilst holding out the hand and using lots of exaggerated repetition and encouragement to get the child to come over
* Ask for the child's cup whilst holding out the hand and using lots of encouraging gestures and looks until the child responds
* Tell the child to sit down whilst pulling out his chair and patting it

* Responding to where the adult is pointing relates to the skill of 'following joint attention', and is an important step in communication development (see Chapter 8).

Routledge
Taylor & Francis Group
ROUTLEDGE

Developing Communicators
Situational understanding

The child begins to respond to **what is said** by learning that when an adult talks:

* A response of some sort is expected and needed (and preferably the one that the adult is after)
* The words are connected to what is going on

However, within this stage, the child still does not understand the individual words; instead, he works out what the adult means from:

* Interpreting the adult's actions, tone of voice and body language
* The familiarity of the situation, because he can use his everyday experiences to predict what the adult wants him to do and what is likely to happen
* The objects, because the child will begin to associate certain objects with certain activities, and this again can help him predict what the adult is likely to be saying

As a result, what is going on is far more important than what is being said. This is referred to as **situational understanding**.

Typical responses during this stage include:

* Responding to a familiar phrase within a familiar situation, for example:
  — 'Do you want a tickle?' and the child starts to squirm and giggle as you bring your hands close to him
  — 'Do you want a kiss?' and the child brings his face close as you lean towards him with your lips
  — 'Let's go to the car', as you are opening the front door, and the child responds by walking out of the door
  — 'Do you want a biscuit?', when you are in the kitchen opening the biscuit tin, and the child responds by racing towards you

The child knows what to do, or what is about to happen, from the actions going on around him, and responds to this.

* Getting a familiar object when asked for as part of an everyday routine, for example responding to:
  — 'Find your shoes', as the adult is putting theirs on
  — 'Where's your book?', when you are in the child's bedroom ready to read his usual night-time story
  — 'Where's your cup?', when you are in the kitchen holding a bottle of milk

Routledge
Taylor & Francis Group
ROUTLEDGE

The child understands what is meant from his familiarity with the routine, and his responses are also triggered by the objects that are used as part of that routine.

* Following a familiar instruction with a familiar object, for example responding to:
  — 'Put this in the bin', as the child is given a sweet wrapper
  — 'Brush your hair', as the child is given his brush

The child understands what is meant by associating those actions with those objects, in those particular situations.

* Turning and coming when called (with lots of encouragement); the child is beginning to recognise the adult's tone of voice when he is required
* Following instructions such as:
  — 'Go to _____' for a familiar person and place (whilst the adult is pointing)
  — 'Give me _____' for an object the child is already holding
  — 'Show me _____' for a familiar part of the body, or an object that the child is already holding (adults generally pick on things that they know the child will respond to, as part of a fun game together)

The child is beginning to recognise and understand these 'run-in' phrases as requiring a specific response, although he relies on the adult's help to be able to complete it, as he may not recognise or understand the word after.

* Pointing to or showing things that are visually obvious and nearby, with lots of clues from the adult; for example the adult might say:
  — 'Where's Daddy?', who is grinning to encourage the child's response
  — 'Where's teddy?', when the child is holding the bear, or it is on the floor, and the adult is looking at it or even touching it to, again, encourage the child's response

Gradually, through the child's experience of hearing the same phrases in the same situations on a regular basis, he begins to recognise the meanings of a few of the most familiar words, which helps him to respond more appropriately to common instructions and phrases around home. However, he would find it very difficult to respond to these same phrases or the individual words outside of these situations.

As a result, throughout this stage, the child's responses to words will be:

* Limited to certain situations and places
* Inconsistent

The child will therefore respond best when he is at home and in his normal routine. Any changes, such as additional people (like Grandma or the speech & language therapist!), or being in a different place (like someone else's home) can mean that the child may not respond – as if the situation is no longer familiar enough to trigger his understanding.

This leads to great frustration and genuine cries of 'But he can do this at home', and to the reassurance that this is typical of this stage of development.

It is not until the next stage that the child can consistently respond and understand the meaning of the word itself, independent from the situation and phrase in which it is used.

Gradually, as this process continues, the child will extract the meaning more and more from what is said and less from what is going on, until finally, at around the four-word level of understanding, the child is able to interpret most of what is said to him from the words, and any misunderstandings can be corrected through further spoken information. See Appendix 1.

Routledge
Taylor & Francis Group
ROUTLEDGE

Understanding first words single-word level   **P-Level**   **P4**

The child begins to understand familiar words independently of the situation or phrase that they are used in. These first words are usually **naming words** (nouns) that are important and significant to the child and have been experienced frequently as part of his well-known routines.

Typically these will relate to:

* Things in the child's routine – bath, teeth, and words relating to changing and dressing
* Things that are used as part of these activities – brush, cup, boots, book
* Things that the child handles and plays with – ball, teddy, shaker
* Things that the child likes – juice, banana, biscuit, cuddle, 'up'
* People and animals in his home – family members and pets

Gradually, as the child learns more about his world and the things that are in it, he expands his understanding of naming words to include more general, but still common and everyday:

* Objects
* People
* Animals
* Places
* Basic everyday action words

During this stage the child is able to pick out and respond to **one** of these words from a simple instruction or phrase.

This stage is referred to as the **single-word level** of comprehension.

As a result of only being able to reliably respond to one word from what has been said, the context is still very significant in helping the child to understand the full meaning of the sentence. For example, two sentences such as 'Where's your car?' and 'Let's go to the car' will both sound like 'car' to a child who can only pick up on one naming word, and his response will be determined by his interpretation of what is going on around him – is the adult looking around the room? Or holding out a hand and walking to the door?

It can be very difficult to formally assess a child at this stage, because his attention control is best when he is involved in his own choice of activity – and not in an adult-directed task (see Chapter 3) and, by their very nature, formal assessments are adult-directed. As a result, the best form of assessment is through the discussion of people's observations within the child's everyday routines at home and school.

So, typical responses that indicate that the child has understood a key word at this point are:

* Anticipatory behaviour of the word that he has picked up on and understood. For example:
  — 'Do you want a tickle?' and the child starts to squirm and giggle before you even move your hands towards him
  — 'Kiss Mummy' and the child moves his face towards you (you may, of course, only actually say 'kiss?', but the key thing is that the child has responded to just the word without you starting to kiss him first)
  — 'Biscuit?' and he races to the kitchen! (Note the difference now that the child does not need to be in the kitchen seeing the tin to be able to respond to what has been said)
  — 'Let's go to the car' and the child goes to the front door before you do

* Following instructions more consistently, and with less encouragement and help. For example:
  — When you tell the child to get his shoes he goes to where they are kept, without your pointing to them
  — If you say 'Find your book' he goes to the lounge and brings it back

* Pointing to things that are visually obvious and nearby, but without the need for the adult to show him first, or encourage his response. For example, the adult might say:
  — 'Where's the ball?', whilst the child is looking at a ball in a picture book
  — 'Where's Daddy?' and now there is no hesitation in pointing to him!
  — Or the adult comments whilst looking in a book, 'I can see a car,' the child goes quiet, looks at the page, then points to the car and gives the adult a big smile!

This page may be photocopied for instructional use only. *The Communication Development Profile* © Charlotte Child 2006

Routledge
Taylor & Francis Group
ROUTLEDGE

Within this stage the child develops a much wider understanding of **action words** (verbs). In addition, during this stage the child begins to be able to pick up and respond to **two key information words** from a simple instruction or phrase.

At first the child will understand and pick up on two:

- **Naming words:**
  - — 'Put the *car* in the *cupboard*'
  - — 'Give the *cup* to *Grandma*'

Later, once the child's understanding of action words is more established, they may use a combination of:

- **Naming and action words:**
  - — '*Throw* the *ball*'
  - — '*Kiss dolly* better'

This stage is referred to as the **two-word level** of comprehension.

The context clearly continues to be very important in helping the child to be able to work out what is expected and to respond appropriately, particularly in longer sentences containing three or four key information words, because the child may only be able to respond reliably to two of these words.

As this stage develops, the child is able to respond to an increasingly wider and more complex vocabulary, including the following.

Negatives

Understanding the combination of 'no' or 'not' and another word, that is to say, that the 'no' affects the other word, for example 'No sweets'. The child generally demonstrates his understanding at this point by protesting!

Questions

- Being able to understand and respond to here-and-now 'where?' questions when the answer is not visually obvious; that is, the child is beginning to respond with new information. For example, the adult asks:
  - — 'Where's pig?' and the child points towards another room
  - — 'Where's the biscuit?' and the child points to his mouth!

- Beginning to link 'what?' with a different type of response, generally giving information about something

Another important development is that the child is beginning to recognise the difference between the way an adult's voice sounds when they are asking a question and when they are telling them to do something, which acts as a big clue as to what response is expected.

Functions

Being able to identify an object indirectly from the description of its use. This is linked to, and dependent upon, understanding action words, for example 'Which one do you eat?' or 'Which one do you sleep in?', when perhaps looking at a picture book or playing in the home corner.

Describing words

* Responding to basic, everyday describing words such as 'gently', 'quiet', 'yucky', 'dirty', 'hot' and 'wait'.

* Responding to functions and describing words signals the beginning of the next stage, 'Understanding describing phrases'.

Established Communicators

Understanding describing phrases
three-word level

Within this stage the child establishes his understanding of basic **describing words**, which at this point are generally:

* Attribute words such as size ('big', 'little', 'small') and colours
* Position words ('in', 'on', 'under', 'up', 'down', 'out')
* Number words ('one', 'lots')

As a rough guide, the describing words that the child will begin to learn and respond to at this stage are ones that are or can be made visually obvious from the context; that is, they refer to features that can be pointed out or reinforced with a gesture as they are said.

More complex words such as time-related vocabulary ('yesterday', 'later', 'wait', 'not now') are notoriously tricky to make the child understand, and are extremely hard to illustrate meaningfully. The child's understanding of these more abstract words therefore develops in the next stage of development – understanding grammar and complex sentences, P7 and P8.

During this stage the child begins to be able to pick up and respond to **three key information words** in a sentence, which now can be combinations of:

* **Naming words**
* **Action words**
* **Describing words**

For example:

* '*Throw* the *ball* to *Molly*'
* '*Put* the *lolly* in the *bag*'
* 'Look, the *red jumper* is in the *basket*'

This is referred to as the **three-word level** of comprehension.

This stage combines the child's knowledge and understanding of things in the world with the language that describes it. For example, when is something big or small? When is it 'under' and not 'in'? What is the difference between long and short, or hot and cold?

The development of language skills within this stage is therefore dependent to some degree on this underlying knowledge of the real world and the child's ability to learn and work things out, that is, his cognitive skills. Further development of vocabulary includes the following.

Negatives

* The child begins to understand longer 'no' and 'not' sentences, and also the forms of 'is not' and 'isn't'. For example:
  — 'That is not yours'
  — 'There are no more biscuits'
  — 'Rabbit isn't here'

* Some children may be able to respond to the full 'is not' form but do not recognise the shortened 'isn't' as having the same meaning until later.

Questions

* Responding to 'what?' and 'where?' questions, which refer to things in the immediate past and future, that is, there are still clues to the answer from within the situation. For example:
  — 'Where's Grandma?' (just after you have waved her off, and the child may point or say 'all gone')
  — 'Where have you been?' (as the child comes in from the garden, and he may point to the garden or say 'garden' or 'bike')
  — 'What did you see?' (just after a lorry passed by)

* The child may also begin to respond to 'Who's this?' questions for very familiar people.

Pronouns

Beginning to be able to work out words that describe the relationship between people:

* I	* My
* Me	* Your
* You	* Mine
* It	* Yours

Within this early stage the adult needs to make the pronoun very obvious and not use it in long phrases — however, the child's response is more likely to be determined by his developing sense of ownership and his reluctance to respond to pronouns relating to others, rather than whether or not he understands it!

This development signals an early understanding of grammatical information and therefore the beginning of the next stage — understanding grammar and complex sentences.

Routledge
Taylor & Francis Group
ROUTLEDGE

Up until this point, the child has been making sense of what has been said through interpreting an increasing range of vocabulary words in simple combinations. Now the child is developing an understanding of **grammar** and how the grammatical information contained in the sentence can change the meaning of the words. The child also begins to follow increasingly more **complex combinations of words**.

During this stage the child begins to be able to pick up and respond to **four or more key information words** in a sentence. These can now be combinations of:

* **Naming words**
* **Action words**
* **Describing words**

and include **grammatical information**.

This stage is referred to as the **four-word level and above**. 'Above' refers to the fact that it is no longer relevant to refer to the number of words that the child is able to listen and respond to, because the significance now shifts to his ability to understand the grammar and more complex forms of sentences.

The P-Level descriptions split this stage of development into:

* P-Level 7: this highlights the ability to follow instructions with four key information words and understand a growing range of more abstract vocabulary, including the more advanced concepts such as time and emotions.

* P-Level 8: this highlights being able to understand grammatical information and the way it changes the meaning of the words and sentences, that is, recognising the difference between past, present and future tenses, singular and plural forms, pronouns, and being able to understand more mature forms of negatives, questions and verbs – to name just the basics.

However, in terms of language development this division is very difficult to make, as the development of understanding of tenses, question forms, pronouns, plurals and other grammatical skills is a continual process across both levels at the same time, and the specific stage of maturity for each level is not stated in the guidance. Therefore, from a speech & language therapy point of view, all skill development within this stage is credited as four-word level and above (ie combining P7 and P8), with the level of maturity of the grammar noted in the assessment description.

The development of understanding of grammar

The following information outlines the key points of grammatical development within each area. Clearly, in terms of assessment, more detailed analysis is needed. However, it provides a useful insight into the amount of grammar that we use in our everyday language, and which – even if we think that we have shortened and simplified the information – how much of it is still far too complex grammatically for children who are in the earlier stages of development.

For example: 'A <u>boy</u> is <u>wash</u>ing the <u>car</u>' (Cavanna, 2003).

In this sentence the core vocabulary words have been underlined, that is, 'boy – wash – car'. The rest can be considered as grammatical information, which is additional words and parts of words that build up around the core vocabulary and provide more specific information relating, for instance, to the timescale, quantities and other concepts (such as place, colour or size) involved.

The meaning of this core sentence can therefore be changed in a number of different ways by adding different bits of grammatical information:

* A boy washed the car (past tense)
* A boy will wash the car (future tense)
* The boys are washing the car (plural)
* The boy is washing her car (pronoun + possession)
* A boy can't wash the car (negative)
* Will a boy wash the car? (question)

Pronouns

The child's understanding of the earlier pronouns becomes more consistent and reliable and he now develops an understanding of the difference between:

* Singular forms: 'he' / 'she', 'him' / 'her'
* Combining with ownership: 'his' / 'her' / 'hers'
* The plural forms: 'they' / 'them' / 'their', then later: 'we' / 'us' / 'our'
* Lastly, the reflexive forms: 'Myself' / 'Yourself', etc

Routledge
Taylor & Francis Group
ROUTLEDGE

Plurals

Being able to understand the difference between singular and plural forms of words. These can be:

* Regular forms with an '-s' or '-es' ending, for example:
  — 'cat' / 'cats'
  — 'house' / 'houses'

* Irregular forms, which involve a whole word change, for example:
  — 'mouse' / 'mice'
  — 'man' / 'men'

Possession

Understanding the use of '-s' at the end of a name indicates ownership, for example, 'That's Molly's'.

Verb tenses

Up until this point the child has been responding to the simple action word; now he is developing his ability to interpret the timescale (tense) from changes to the word endings or to the whole word:

* Present tense: understanding that the '-ing' form is telling you about an action that is happening there and then, for example, 'Florence is jumping high'

* Past tense: understanding both:
  — Irregular forms, where the whole word changes, eg 'eat' / 'ate'
  — Regular forms, with the addition of '-ed', eg 'walk' / 'walked'

* Future tense: the child needs to be able to pick up and understand the use of words such as:
  — 'Going to'
  — 'Will'
  — 'Shall'

Learning about future tenses is very much harder because it involves having to think about and understand something that has not yet happened – but will do. It is also all caught up with learning those all-too-important and frustrating words such as 'not now', 'later' and 'wait'.

* Complex verbs: the child also expands his understanding of action words to include ones which imply a condition or mood, and he therefore begins to understand more abstract, hidden meanings:
  — Have (got to)   — Should
  — Must   — Might
  — Would   — Ought
  — Could

Negatives

* This now changes from being able to understand simple combinations of 'no' and 'not' in a sentence to the child beginning to develop his understanding of negative-word vocabulary, including:
  — 'Cannot'/'Can't'   — 'Won't'
  — 'Do not'/'Don't'   — 'Must not'/'Mustn't'

* Then the past tense versions:
  — 'Did not'/'didn't'   — 'Has not'/'hasn't'

* And, later on, combined with the conditional tenses too:
  — 'Couldn't'   — 'Wasn't'
  — 'Wouldn't'

Questions

The child begins to respond to more abstract questions that rely on him fully understanding the vocabulary used.

* 'Where?' and 'what?' questions that ask about the less immediate past and future, and about things where there are few, if any, visual or situational clues. For example:
  — 'Where are we going with Sophie?'
  — 'Who is coming for tea?'
  — 'Where did Molly go with her mum?'

* The child's understanding of question-word vocabulary expands to include:
  — How?   — Which?
  — Why?   — How many/much?
  — When?

Routledge
Taylor & Francis Group
ROUTLEDGE

The development of understanding of complex sentences

A sentence can be described as a **complex sentence** if:

* It contains four or more information words
* It contains grammatical information
* It contains more than one main action word ('Mummy *is going to see* her friends')
* It is made up of two phrases linked by 'and', 'because' or 'to' / 'in order to' (as there is the need to understand the sequence or cause-and-effect information it implies, eg 'Nell is happy because it's her party')
* The 'is being' form is used (because the sequence of words becomes different from the sequence of events, and needs skill in holding the information and working out who has done what to whom, eg 'The horse is being sat on by Verity' – meaning the same as 'Verity is sitting on the horse')

With so much verbal information in a sentence it is easy for the child to become overloaded. The number of words that he can follow will be affected at first by the additional amount of grammatical information that the sentence contains.

Gradually the child becomes better at sorting out the information and can then begin to interpret longer and more complex sentences reliably.

However, for a child who has any difficulty with sequencing, organising and remembering what was said, even if his understanding of all the individual words is good, it will still be very difficult for him to work out the meaning of complex sentences.

Describing words

The complexity of the general words that the child can understand becomes more abstract and defines more and more subtle differences, most of which are concepts that are very hard to visualise or represent visually when talking to the child, which makes them much harder to learn and understand. For example:

* Quality (hard, smooth, rough, different, tight)
* Quantity (full, empty, without, a little)
* Emotions (happy, sad, curious, excited)
* Size (shallow, thin, high, thick)
* Time (first, next, later, before, after)
* Position (behind, in front, next to, between)

Routledge P
Taylor & Francis Group
ROUTLEDGE

The above are only illustrative examples; for a more detailed evaluation of concept words see assessments such as the Bracken *Basic Concept Scale – Revised* (1998).

As well as being able to work out the meaning of a sentence from the words and grammar used, the child also needs to develop skills in *interpreting all the unspoken messages* that we give through our body language, facial expressions and tone of voice, even noticing the adult's level of interest or listening.

One example is **inference**: we have all been there … the doorbell rings and a voice from the bathroom shouts 'I'm in the bath.' On the face of it, the words bear little relationship to the situation, but the unspoken or inferred meaning is, 'I can't get to the door – can you answer it?'

This is an enormously important ability that we rely on a lot as adults, because it allows us to miss out having to actually say all the additional information of 'I've just this moment got into the bath and now there is someone at the door – please can you give me five minutes' peace and answer it!'

So, if a child can only interpret the words that you say and not the contextual information, he is described as having 'literal understanding'.

Another example is in understanding **sarcasm**, which involves interpreting the meaning of the words in relation to the situation and the speaker's manner.

Consider the following scenarios where the phrase 'Oh, fantastic' is used:

* Whilst looking at your brand new car

* Whilst looking at your brand new car, just after someone has backed into it

* Whilst looking at your brand new car, just after someone has backed into it and driven off without exchanging insurance details!

Understanding these 'higher language skills' is not covered in depth in this Profile. although some reference is made to them in Chapter 8, which deals with conversational skills.

Expression
How the child communicates

Communication between a parent and child can be considered to start from birth. Within hours relatives are heard to say 'Oh look, he is hungry', or tired, or uncomfortable, or in pain, and all of these judgements come from the adult interpreting the child's behaviours and reactions. As a result the child's expressive language development can be observed in the Early Communicators phase as the development of communicative behaviours. This begins with the way the child reacts and responds to things going on around and within him, and eventually to the development of planned and purposeful actions that initially help him to get things done for himself and later are directed at adults in order for them to do things for him. Finally, in the Developing Communicators phase, these behaviours are replaced by more recognisable forms of communication such as gestures, vocalisations and words.

'Expression' in this Profile refers to the development of a shared communication system, that is, one that is understandable and used by others. Therefore all reference to language and words includes the use of speech, writing, signing, gestures, symbols, pictures, photos, objects of reference and voice output communication aids (VOCAs), in any combination.

The change from the child using communicative behaviours to more conventional forms of communication, using any system, involves the development of a number of different skills:

* The range of words that the child can use (naming, action, describing words)
* The number of words that the child can put together
* The amount of grammatical information that he can use
* His ability to organise and sequence words – to make longer and more complex sentences, but still manages to say what he means
* Being able to use non-verbal communication to convey meaning appropriately
* The sound system – which is considered in its own chapter

The development of these skills is underpinned by:

* The child's understanding of the words (comprehension)
* And what the words refer to in the real world (cognitive skills)

Routledge
Taylor & Francis Group
ROUTLEDGE

A child's spoken language skills can break down within any one, or a combination of, these areas, and cause significant difficulties.

How do you Work Out the Child's 'Word Level' for his Spoken Language Skills?

Speech & language therapists count the number of words that the child uses in a sentence to give the word level.

> The word level for the child's spoken language skills equals the number of words that the child puts together in a single sentence.

For example, if a child says:

* 'dog' = one-word level
* 'dog ball' = two-word level
* 'dog ball mouth' = three-word level
* 'dog got ball in mouth' = four-word level and above (you do not continue to count beyond four words)

In this way 'key' words are not identified or counted.

The P-Level descriptions, however, are based upon key words, as follows:

* P-Level 6 expects combinations of any three words, eg 'Me want muffin' (ie equivalent to three-word level).

* P-Level 7 gives examples of combinations of four or more words (ie equivalent to four-word level) with up to three key vocabulary words, eg 'I want a chocolate muffin.'

* P-Level 8 expects combinations of four or more words, with up to four key vocabulary words, eg 'I want a big chocolate muffin.'

However, even in these examples from the QCA guidelines, it is arguable as to what the 'key' words are — and how they are defined, which is why speech & language therapists focus at that point (P7 and P8), on the way vocabulary words, grammatical words and parts of words combine to form sentences — as a way of assessing a child's language level.

Finally, although it is often easier to observe and judge a child's expressive language skills from what you hear him say, it is very important to ensure you have a clear assessment of his comprehension levels and his cognitive skills, too, as this informs you about how much the child really understands of what he is saying.

Routledge — Taylor & Francis Group — This page may be photocopied for instructional use only. *The Communication Development Profile* © Charlotte Child 2006

Expression – Overview of Developmental Stages

Early Communicators		P-LEVEL
* INVOLUNTARY REACTIONS AND REFLEXES		**P1(i) and P1(ii)**
* VOLUNTARY REACTIONS		**P2(i)**
* 'IF I DO … I GET …'		**P2(ii)**
* 'IF I DO … YOU DO …'		**P3(i)**
Developing Communicators		
* SITUATIONAL COMMUNICATION		**P3(ii)**
* USING FIRST WORDS	*Single-word level*	**P4**
* USING SIMPLE PHRASES	*Two-word level*	**P5**
Established Communicators		
* USING DESCRIBING PHRASES	*Three-word level*	**P6**
* USING GRAMMAR AND COMPLEX SENTENCES		**P7 and P8**
	Four-word level and above	

Each of these stages is explained in detail on pages 62–81.

Early Communicators

Involuntary reactions and reflexes *Involuntary reactions and reflexes* **P-Levels** **P1(i) and P1(ii)**

The child has a small range of movements and behaviours, which are **involuntary reactions or reflexes**, that is, not under his control; for example:

* Crying
* Squirming
* Changes in colour
* Startle reflex
* Going quiet
* Looking
* Noises
* Level of wakefulness

Voluntary reactions

The child is able to produce a wider range of movements and behaviours, which are now **voluntary reactions**, that is, the child can control their use; for example:

* Smiling
* Turning
* Noises/vocalisations
* Looking
* Holding things
* Moving legs and arms (and other body movements)

Within simple, repetitive games the adult, often without realising it, creates pauses for the child to 'have a go' with their noises or movements, but maintains the structure by carrying on if the child does not respond.

In this stage of communicative development the child begins to explore and create changes in his immediate environment through **planned and purposeful actions**.

First, the child is learning that if he does this ... then that happens, which can also be described as 'If I do ... I get ...'. Typical examples include:

* Looking and reaching towards something that has fallen out of his grasp
* Trying to get to something that is out of reach
* Trying to make something work
* Exploring an object
* Taking an offered item from the adult

This 'having a go' can be called 'I know what I want' intentional behaviour or 'goal-directed behaviour', as the child knows what he wants and goes for it, but does not try to involve the adult. In fact, usually the adult only becomes aware that the child is trying to reach something or do something when they see or hear his efforts, or hear his cry of frustration and anger because he cannot do it. See Chapter 4 for a fuller description and criteria for 'I know what I want' intentional behaviour.

Second, the child also begins to respond very purposefully when certain things happen, for example:

* Screaming when something or someone goes out of sight
* Making excited movements as he sees his food or drink being prepared
* Making noises as he is trying to do something

The most important planned and purposeful action is the development of the **'reach-for-real'**, that is, the child looking and reaching for an item that he wants.

* Initially, this action will be looking and reaching towards something that has simply fallen out of the child's grasp
* Later, the child will let go of one toy to pick up and look at another one that is in reach
* Finally, he will reach towards a toy that is out of reach and, rather than immediately giving up, will keep trying to get it for himself

The significance in terms of communication development is that this last example is the first real action that the adult is able to clearly attach a meaning to, and it acts as a big signal to the adult of 'I want that'. As a result, the adult, providing they have noticed, responds by picking the item up and handing it over, generally with some sort of comment, 'Here you are, here's your monkey,' and from that, the child begins to experience that the adult can respond and do things for them.

This page may be photocopied for instructional use only. *The Communication Development Profile* © Charlotte Child 2006

Routledge
Taylor & Francis Group

ROUTLEDGE

In addition, during this stage, the adult becomes far more selective about the behaviours that are recognised as being 'communicative', and is much more likely to respond and 'read a message' when the child is either:

* Looking
* Reaching
* Making noises

This, in turn, encourages the child to use these successful behaviours even more, and gradually to replace his use of the earlier ones.

Routledge
Taylor & Francis Group
ROUTLEDGE

In this stage the child begins to make things happen through others, using his behaviours and actions as **communication strategies**.

He is starting to learn that if he does this ... an adult does that. This can therefore be called 'If I do ... You do ...', because the child is beginning to involve the adult in achieving his goal, rather than doing it for himself. Typically these behaviours will include:

The child acting directly on the adult:

* Pulling the adult to things, for example the door handle so the child can go out
* Putting the adult's hand on things, for example a toy the child wants to make work
* Bringing things over for the adult to look at

The child's own actions:

* Using the whole body, for example going rigid or floppy
* Pushing things away or turning away from something
* Looking towards something he wants
* Reaching towards something he wants
* Purposeful screaming and making noises

This change to directing behaviours at another person marks a shift from the previous 'I know what I want' intentional behaviour, to the beginnings of 'I'm telling you what I want' intentional communicative behaviour. See Chapter 4 for a fuller description and criteria.

An important indicator of this change is when the earlier 'reach-for-real', in which the child gets an item for himself, is gradually replaced by the **'reach-for-signal'**, that is, the child reaching towards something he wants whilst making purposeful (often protesting) noises at it, therefore gaining the adult's attention and making it quite clear that he wants something to happen (although it may not be clear what this is!).

Routledge
Taylor & Francis Group
ROUTLEDGE

It must be remembered that this is the early stage of intentional communication and the child is only just learning how to gain and direct an adult's attention. As a result, these initial attempts at communicating are still very hit and miss, with the child using behavioural strategies that are:

* Easily missed, so if the adult does not notice his behaviours, the moment is usually lost because, in this early stage, the child does not persist with his attempts to communicate
* Uncoordinated, with the child directing his behaviours either at the adult or towards what he wants to get or do, but not pulling this together
* Difficult to interpret, with the adult only knowing that they have got it right when the child finally goes quiet and is happy

This leads to many abandoned attempts and lots of frustration all round!

Developing Communicators

'And I Won't Give Up!'
use of situational communication

There are two important developments within this stage: first, the child begins to convey his messages by using far more sophisticated and recognisable combinations of **communicative behaviours**:

* Gestures
* Vocalisations
* Protowords
* First words

Second, the child is really taking on the responsibility for getting a message across for himself by being very persistent in his use of these behaviours, hence the term 'If I do … You do … And I won't give up'. As a result the child's communication skills are now considered to be fully intentional. (See Chapter 4 for a fuller description of, and criteria for, 'I'm telling you what I want' intentional communicative behaviours.)

However, within this stage the child's use of these communication behaviours continues to be highly dependent on what is going on around him and the prompts that this provides; for example, the range of situations that these behaviours are used in is limited, often only to food or drink and about where the child wants to be (for example, in or out of his chair or the room), or for attention.

The behaviours may only be triggered by being in specific situations and the same behaviours may not be used to request a different item, or even the same item in a different situation. Therefore, the child may request in one way at home and differently at school, or inconsistently across the day.

The child's attempts are usually triggered by things that are in sight, for example a banana or the car keys on the table – his communication is very much about the 'here and now'.

So the child's use of these new strategies will still be:

* Limited to certain situations and places
* Inconsistent

This stage is referred to as the **use of situational communication**.

As a result, the child's communication skills are still very fragile, and he will revert to a bombardment of the earlier behaviours in order to make his needs known if his attempts fail the first time. For this reason it is also very important at this stage to focus on the development of the messages that the child is beginning to communicate, because the development of *why* he is communicating becomes much more significant as a measure of progress than *how* he is communicating – as this can remain the same and situation-specific for some time (see Chapter 8).

Gestures which convey meaning include:

* Nodding/shaking the head
* Waving
* Holding out the hand – as a request to be given something
* Holding out an object (but not letting go) – to show it
* Holding and giving an object
* Pointing
* Personalised gestures made up by the child (that only the most familiar people can interpret)

(Note the 'reach-for-signal' becomes a more sophisticated point; further development comes with the distance from the child to what they are referring to.)

Vocalisations refer to the range of sounds and noises that a child uses, sometimes to himself and sometimes to help him communicate a message. Their combination with a gesture marks a shift towards more sound-based communication.

Protowords are the child's very first attempts to convey a specific meaning through a consistent pattern of sounds, but they can also have multiple uses. For example, 'doh' may mean 'dog', 'cuddle' or 'ball', but its meaning at that moment will hopefully be clear from the context. Some protowords may not have an identifiable meaning but are used consistently in certain situations, such as my own daughter saying 'gellar gellar' whenever she saw the dogs out in the garden – she clearly knew what she meant, but we do not to this day!

First words develop from the protowords; they are more easily identifiable as being words with a more specific meaning and pattern of use. However, they are still best understood by familiar people and within a known context. Within this situational stage there will only be a very limited number of what could reliably be described as 'first words'. Their development only really gets going within the next stage ('Using first words'), when the child's understanding and use of words and what they mean becomes independent from what is going on around him.

The child begins to establish his use of his first words, predominantly **naming words** (nouns), to label and refer to things in his immediate environment, and also a range of words which evolve from the messages that he wants to communicate.

Typically, these first words will be related to:

* Things in the child's routine – bath, teeth, car, juice, biscuit
* Things that the child likes and wants – different foods and drinks
* Games and places the child wants to be (eg 'baa' for 'Baa Baa Black Sheep', 'up' to get a cuddle or to avoid walking and 'out' from the highchair or room)
* People and animals in the child's home – family members, pets
* Happening words – 'no', 'hiya', 'bye', 'look', 'Mummy', 'Daddy'*

* The words 'Mummy' and 'Daddy' have been put under 'happening words' because they are first used to call for attention rather than to refer specifically to the person. This is a good illustration of how a child's use of communication begins to influence and lead his language learning. Chapter 6 focusses on the technical development of words and word combinations, deliberately separating this skill from what can be considered as the driving force of communicative development – why the child is communicating and what he is communicating about. This is covered in Chapter 8.

Gradually, as the child learns more about his world and the things that are in it, he expands his use of these words to refer to and name more general:

* Objects
* People
* Animals
* Places

Within this stage the child gets his message across by using a **single word** along with a range of communicative behaviours such as pointing, reaching and vocalisation.

This is referred to as the **single-word level** of expression.

There is also development in the situations in which the child uses the word which indicates the level of independence the child is at with selecting and using words:

* After the adult has said it, eg adult: 'Here's your apple' and the child spontaneously copies 'apple', as he takes it. Or, in the bath, when the parent says 'Look, bubbles' and the child says 'bubbles' after them
* When he can see it, eg the apple is in a bowl on the table, the child walks over, starts to reach towards it whilst saying 'apple?'. Or when the child gets into the bath he says 'bubbles' as he begins to splash about

Routledge
Taylor & Francis Group
ROUTLEDGE

* When the item is out of sight, eg the child is in a different room from the fruit bowl, looks at the adult and says 'apple?'. Or after the parent has said that it is time for a bath, the child says 'bubbles?'.

This last use is the most sophisticated as it indicates a firmly established link between the item and the word that refers to it, as the child has not needed any visual prompt to come up with the word. However, the child's use of words will still be situation-dependent to some extent throughout this stage, because different places have different things in them and also different communicative needs and demands.

The child may routinely use words at home to ask for things and draw attention to something of interest, but at nursery or school he may only communicate through earlier non-speaking behaviours – much to his parents' despair and yet more genuine cries of 'But he can say that at home!' I know – I've been there and have a very big T-shirt for this experience! The inconsistency is simply part of this stage, and reduces as the child's skills become more established and independent.

The context and the child's use of his earlier communicative behaviours (such as gestures, crying or pulling etc) continue to be very important in helping the adult to work out the meaning of the child's message, and it follows that the child is still best understood by people who are the most familiar with him and the things that he usually communicates about within a given situation. For example, screaming and reaching and saying 'bah bah' at a mealtime may convey all the meaning that a parent needs to produce a banana whilst Grandma watches with a bemused look! However, those same behaviours as the bath is running will result in the child being hastily undressed and put in.

In addition, the child's determination and persistence in making sure that he is heard and understood, and that he gets what he wants, remain very significant in his success as a communicator, and are important skills which need to develop continually.

The child begins to put **two words** together. Typical early combinations include:

* '_____ please'
* 'More _____'
* 'Hello_____'
* 'Bye bye _____'
* 'All gone _____'
* '_____ look'

The child also begins to establish a range of **action words** (verbs) and an increasing and more consistent use of naming words in response to more and more abstract situations and materials. As a result later phrases are combinations of:

* **Naming words** and/or
* **Action words**
  — 'Dog garden'
  — 'Ball Nell'
  — 'Daddy shoe'
  — 'Mummy laugh'
  — 'Clap hands'

(At this stage the child does not necessarily put an '-ing' on the action words.)

This stage is referred to as the **two-word level** of expression.

The context clearly continues to play a very important role in helping the adult to work out what the child means. For example, if a child says, 'Mummy shoe' it could mean:

* 'That's Mummy's shoe' (statement)
* 'I want Mummy's shoe' (request)
* 'Where is Mummy's shoe?' (question)
* 'Put on your shoe Mummy!' (instruction)

It is also very important that the child gains skills in using his language skills to communicate for all of those reasons in brackets, and therefore that his targets are not just based on teaching word combinations but also for a range of intentions. (See Chapter 8 for a further discussion of this and an assessment framework.)

Routledge
Taylor & Francis Group
ROUTLEDGE

Further development of vocabulary and sentence structure includes the following:

Negatives

These begin to develop through the use of a single word 'no' to mean:

* 'I don't want to' (refusing for himself)
* 'Don't do that' (stopping someone else from doing it)
* 'No it isn't' (denying, also known as being awkward!)
* 'Can't do it' (communicating an inability to do something)

Questions

There are two types of questions, and they develop in parallel:

* Those which start with a question word. The first to develop are 'What' and Where', in two-word combinations, where the second word is either a simple noun or non-specific 'this' or 'that', for example:
  — 'Where Mummy?'
  — 'What that?'

* Intonation questions, that is, those which tend to have a yes/no answer and a distinctive rise and fall in the speaker's voice. Again, at this point these consist of two-word combinations, for example:
  — 'Dog walk?'
  — 'Go out?'
  — 'Boots on?'

Functions

Being able to describe an object indirectly by what it is used for, which links to the child's development of his action word vocabulary. For example, whilst looking at an apple and asked about what it is used for, the child replies, 'eat it', or for a chair as 'sit' or 'sit down'. This is obviously limited to very simple explanations and associations at this point.

Describing words

Use of basic, everyday describing words through association with the situation. These words may be used on their own or with another naming word. For example, 'yucky', 'dirty', 'hot', 'sticky', 'wet', 'hurt', 'naughty', 'cross', and combined in simple phrases: 'sticky fingers', 'dog wet', 'red car', 'in there', 'too tight', 'naughty dog', 'Mummy cross'.

The development of a describing word vocabulary signals the start of the next stage, 'Using describing phrases.'

Routledge P
Taylor & Francis Group
ROUTLEDGE

Established Communicators

Using describing phrases *three-word level*

The child's **describing word vocabulary** expands rapidly. Generally it includes:

* Attribute words such as size ('big', 'little', 'small') and colour
* Position words ('in', 'on', 'under', 'up', 'down', 'out')
* Number words ('one', 'lots')

A rough rule to the development of the child's descriptive vocabulary at this point is that the words will generally relate to observable features that can be easily pointed out, or reinforced using a simple gesture. Words such as 'yesterday', 'love' or 'funny', for instance, are more abstract and very difficult to show visually – these are the sort of words that develop in the next stage as the child's language skills become more internalised.

In addition, the child also begins to use sentences containing **three words**, which can now be combinations of:

* **Naming words**
* **Action words**
* **Describing words**

This stage is referred to as the **three-word level** of expression.

It is important to note that speech & language therapists refer to a three-word-level sentence as being a sentence made up of a combination of any three words; it does not matter whether the words are 'key words' or not. (See the overview of expression earlier in this chapter for a fuller explanation.)

Further development of vocabulary and sentence structure includes the following.

Action words

* The child starts to put '-ing' on the end of the verb (but not consistently)
* He uses 'do' as a simple, unspecific action word, for example:
  — 'Robyn laughing'
  — 'Daddy do it'

Negatives

* These involve using simple combinations of 'no' or 'not' and up to three other words, where the negative words stay outside the phrase, for example 'No sleep', 'No shoes', 'No Foh-Foh do it' (where the child is referring to himself).
* This then changes with the 'no' and 'not' inside the phrase, for example, 'I not want to', 'Foh-Foh not sleep'.

This page may be photocopied for instructional use only. *The Communication Development Profile* © Charlotte Child 2006

Questions

In general, the child is asking questions about things in the 'here and now', but which may not be in sight, and about things in the immediate past and future.

Question words:

* 'Where' and 'what' combined with two other words, but still not action words; for example:
  — 'What that for?'
  — 'Where my shoes?'

* The use of 'where' and 'what' in set phrases using the unspecific action words 'do' and 'go', such as 'where' + 'go/going/gone', and 'what' + 'do/doing/done'; for example:
  — 'Where daddy gone?'
  — 'What Verity doing?'

* The use of 'who' in set phrases, for example:
  — 'Who this?'
  — 'Who that?'

Intonation questions:

* These now consist of three-word combinations, for example:
  — 'Go dog walk?'
  — 'Daddy dog walk?'

Early grammar

This point involves the rather inconsistent use of:

* Grammatical words, such as 'the' and 'a' in sentences, although in fact these are likely to appear at first as extra sounds between the words rather than a deliberate attempt to say them individually.

* Pronouns:
  — I
  — Me
  — You
  — It
  — My
  — Your
  — Mine
  — Yours

  The use of these pronouns is being driven by the child's preoccupation with ownership – particularly relating to his claims on other people's possessions!

The development of this early grammar and the use of four-word phrases signals the onset of the next stage, 'Using grammar and complex sentences'.

Up until this point the child has been using simple combinations of information words, and their sentences will have sounded rather like a telegram. Now the child begins to use **longer and more complex sentences** containing **grammatical information**.

The child's sentences are typically 4–8 words long and can include a much more extensive range of word combinations, including the key ones, of:

* **Naming words**
* **Action words**
* **Describing words**

and **grammatical information**.

This stage is therefore referred to as the **four-word level and above**. ('Above' refers to the fact that the significance now shifts from noting the number of vocabulary words that the child can use, to his ability to use grammar and more complex forms of sentences.)

The P-Level descriptions split the four-word level stage of development into two separate ones according to the number of key vocabulary words.

P-Level 7 outlines the use of:

* Four or more words in a sentence, containing up to three key words
* The development of grammar, specifically tenses and plurals
* Linking sentences with 'and'

P-Level 8 outlines the use of longer and more complex sentences with:

* Four or more words in a sentence, containing four or more key words
* The development of a wider range of vocabulary, including the use of more advanced concepts such as time and emotions
* The ongoing development of grammar, specifically possessives
* Linking sentences with 'because' / ''cos'

However, this division is very difficult to make, as the development of tenses, question forms, pronouns, plurals and other grammatical skills is a continual process across both levels at the same time, and the specific stage of maturity for each level is not stated in the guidance. Therefore, from a speech & language therapy point of view, all skill development within this stage is credited as four-word level and above (ie combining P7 and P8), with the level of maturity of the grammar noted in the assessment description.

This page may be photocopied for instructional use only. The Communication Development Profile © Charlotte Child 2006

Routledge
Taylor & Francis Group
ROUTLEDGE

The development of use of grammar

The following information outlines the key points of grammatical development within each area and will help to identify the child's pattern of use.

Pronouns

The child's use of the pronouns outlined in 'Using describing phrases' (three-word level) becomes more reliable and consistent, and he now begins to develop his use of:

* Singular forms, 'he' / 'she', 'him' / 'her'
* Combining with ownership, 'his' / 'her' / 'hers'
* Plural forms, 'they' / 'them' / 'their' and 'we' / 'us' / 'our'
* Reflexive forms, 'myself' / 'yourself' etc

Plurals

These include the development of the use of:

* Regular forms with an '-s' or '-es' ending, for example:
  — 'cat' / 'cats'
  — 'house' / 'houses'
* Irregular forms, which involve a whole word change, for example:
  — 'mouse' / 'mice'
  — 'man' / 'men'

Possession

Developing the use of '-s' at the end of a word to confirm ownership, for example: 'That not yours, it Daisy's', 'It mines'.

Verb tenses

Up until this point the child has been using phrases with a single main action word with or without '-ing' on the end, and all in the 'here and now' present tense. Now, along with the development of the child's understanding of time and time concepts, there is an expansion in the different forms of verbs that the child can use, which help to inform us about the timescale.

Present tense – this expands to include:

* A more established use of '-ing' *and*
* The use of the third person singular '-s' at the end of the verb, for example:
  — 'Thomas is swimming'
  — 'Florence likes ice cream'
  — 'Agatha walks to the shop'

This page may be photocopied for instructional use only. *The Communication Development Profile* © Charlotte Child 2006

Routledge
Taylor & Francis Group
ROUTLEDGE

Past tense:

*   This often starts off with the use of a non-specific general word, such as 'been' and 'done', to signal that an activity has happened, for example:
    — 'I been dog walk'
    — 'I done eat banana'

*   Irregular forms, which involve a whole word change, for example:
    — 'Thomas swam'

*   Regular forms where '-ed' is added to the end, for example:
    — 'Agatha walked to the shops'

The use of '-ed' on the end is usually over-generalised at first, for example, 'I goed to the shops', 'Thomas swammed'.

Auxiliaries:

The use of a second bit of the action word (also known as an auxiliary verb), which adds further meaning and structure to the sentence, and can be singular or plural, and in the present tense or past tense:

*   'am'   *   'was'
*   'are'   *   'were'
*   'is'

The extra part of the verb can either confirm the main verb in terms of the tense and person involved, for example:

*   'I am jumping'
*   'Nell was running'
*   'Kit and Robert are climbing'

Or it can provide the timescale and override the action word form, for example:

*   'I was jumping'
*   'Nell was running'
*   'Kit and Robert were climbing'

Future tense:

This starts off with a general, non-specific use of 'going to' / 'gonna' to show that the action has not happened yet. At first it will be used as the child is about to embark on the task, 'I gonna feed teddy', and then later to talk about the more distant future, 'I going dog walk morning'.

*   Will – appears later
*   Shall – appears later

Routledge P This page may be photocopied for instructional use only. The Communication Development Profile © Charlotte Child 2006

Complex verbs – the use of action words that convey a mood or a condition:

* Have (got to)
* Must
* Would
* Could

* Should
* Might
* Ought

Negatives

Changes from adding 'no' and 'not' to a sentence, to the development and use of negative word vocabulary:

* The use, singly or in simple set phrases, of:
    — 'can't'/'can't do it'
    — 'don't'/'don't do it'
    — 'won't'/'won't do it'

* Their combinations with specific verbs:
    — 'don't like it'
    — 'can't see it'
    — 'won't eat it'

* Use of past tense forms:
    — 'did not'/'didn't'
    — 'couldn't'/'wouldn't'
    — 'haven't'/'hasn't'
    — 'wasn't'

Questions

The child begins to ask more abstract questions, which are about the less immediate past and future, and about things where there are few, if any, visual or situational clues.

Question words

* The use of 'where' and 'what' combined with specific verbs, for example:
    — 'What Daddy eating?'
    — 'Where Verity running?'

* The question word vocabulary now expands to include the use of:
    — How
    — Why
    — When
    — Which
    — How many/much

Intonation questions

The sentences become very much longer and start to begin with 'Can you ...', or 'Are you ...' or 'Do you ...', for example:
— 'Can I have a biscuit?'
— 'Are you going dog walk?'
— 'Is Annie coming for tea?'

Tag questions

Tag questions also begin to emerge, and literally involve the child tagging an intonation question on to the end of a sentence. They are usually used in order to get a confirmation of something and for this reason often seem to be accompanied by that pleading look! They generally start with a simple 'OK?' on the end, for example:

❋ 'I get a biscuit, OK?'

And then use a range of different forms, for example:

❋ 'That big fishes, aren't they?'

Grammatical words

The use of 'little' words such as 'the', 'a', 'to' and 'of' become more consistent and deliberate. These are words which do not have a specific meaning on their own but, when combined with a vocabulary word, add to and refine the overall meaning, and play an important part in making the sentence sound more mature and coherent, and less 'telegrammatic'.

The development of the use of longer and more complex sentences

A sentence can be described as a **complex sentence** if it contains:

❋ Four or more information words
❋ Grammatical information
❋ More than one main action word, eg 'Mummy was wanting to go to the shops'

In addition, sentences become longer and more complex through the use of **connecting words**:

❋ By linking together two naming words or phrases, for example:
— 'I eat my banana and my yoghurt'
— 'I got my hat and my yellow gloves'

* By linking together two simple phrases (each with their own action words), for example:
  — 'Sophie was running and she fell over'
  — 'You sit here and I'll sit there'

* By linking with words that tell you about the 'cause and effect' relationship of the actions, for example:
  — 'Sophie is crying because she fell over'
  — 'Robyn is running to catch the ball'

Describing words

The sentences also become more complex as the child begins to use more abstract words that define more and more subtle differences. As a rough guide, at this point these are features or concepts that are very hard to show visually, and can only really be explained through using more language – which makes them much harder to learn and use. For example:

* Quality (hard, smooth, rough, different, tight)
* Quantity (full, empty, without, a little)
* Emotions (happy, sad, curious, excited)
* Size (shallow, thin, high, thick)
* Time (first, next, later, before, after)
* Position (behind, in front, next to, between)

The above are only illustrative examples; for a more detailed evaluation of concept words see assessments such as the Bracken (1998) and PORIC (Woods & Acors, 1999).

There are clearly a lot of additional skills beyond just these language-based ones which the child now needs to learn in order to be able to communicate even more effectively. Those that relate to the child's use of his language skills, such as inference and prediction, are covered in Chapter 8.

Other skills, often referred to as the 'higher language skills', such as the development of reasoning and being able to organise and sequence information (and therefore express increasingly more complex and abstract ideas), are not considered in depth in this Profile.

Sound System Development

The following table outlines the general pattern of development of a child's sound system in terms of the emergence and use of the sounds in words. It helps to identify the broad range of sounds that you would expect to see developing in relation to the child's language development, and in this way, indicates whether or not the child's sound system is particularly delayed or simply reflects his overall stage of language development. This table does not identify the pattern of use for each individual sound and this level of assessment would need to be undertaken by a speech & language therapist.

Early Communicators

Play at making sounds and noises.

Whilst changes to a child's vocal production can be seen during these stages, they are not relevant to planning at this stage.

Developing Communicators

SITUATIONAL COMMUNICATION	P3(ii)	Using sounds and noises to mean things.					
FIRST WORDS	P4	Using sounds in early words; very variable patterns.					
SIMPLE PHRASES	P5	m	n	p	b	t	d

Established Communicators

DESCRIBING PHRASES	P6	k	g	ng	f	s		
GRAMMAR and COMPLEX SENTENCES	P7 and P8	v	z	sh	ch	j	th	zh
		h	w	r	l	y		

Clusters (s)	sp	st	sk	sm	sn	sl	sw	
Clusters (l)	pl	bl	kl	gl	fl			
Clusters (r)	pr	br	tr	dr	kr	gr	fr	thr
Clusters (w)	tw	kw						
	skw	str	spr					

Note

'ng' as in 'ri**ng**'/'j' as in '**j**am', 'ba**dge**'/'zh' as in 'mea**s**ure'

Adapted from Grunwell (1982)

Sound System Development

Use of Communication Skills
What and why the child communicates

For a child to be able to communicate effectively and independently, without having to rely on an adult noticing and interpreting his behaviours, or to rely on being asked 'do you want' questions, he needs to be able to start an interaction and then direct the adult's attention to what he wants them to do or what he wants them to look at.

In order to communicate, a child also needs:

* A message worth communicating about, by his standards – not the adults (ie what and why he is communicating)

* An opportunity to give the message (ie where, when and with whom)

* A way of communicating the message (that can be understood by others)

Money and Thurman (1994)

For example, if a child has something he is very motivated to communicate about and has an opportunity to give his message, he will generally find a way of doing so, even if it does mean a behavioural meltdown.

However, it does not necessarily work the other way round; just because a child has a range of words and phrases does not mean that he will use them to communicate a message.

The previous chapters have described the development of comprehension (what the child understands) and expression (how the child communicates), and how they contribute to the child's ability to communicate. This chapter focusses on the way that the child uses these skills to communicate, and what and why he communicates.

Routledge
Taylor & Francis Group
ROUTLEDGE

As children begin to learn their first words there is an instinctive move by adults towards teaching them new ones, and in particular the names of the things and people around them. Whilst this helps in developing the child's understanding of these words it does not provide the motivation to use them. An all too familiar situation occurs when the adult asks 'What's that?', and the child gives you the look of 'You know it's a dog, I know it's a dog – so why do I have to say it's a dog?' followed inevitably by silence!

The first things that children start to tell us about are the people, things, animals, events and situations in their lives which have importance and meaning to them.

For example: when you see the rather large family cat walk past, you point it out to your child and say 'cat', and you do the same when you see a cat in the street, at someone else's house, in books and on television. One day your child sees the cat walk into the room, points and says 'dah'; you are delighted – he has learnt the word 'cat' (at last). However, your child does not then point to any other cat you encounter and you are frustrated that it seemed a one-off.

One reason for this, and there are many, is in fact that your child was not saying 'Hey, look, there's a cat [a furry feline that likes milk and mice]' but 'Hey, look, I know what that is and it lives in my house.' The child is communicating what the situation means to him rather than labelling the things involved.

These communication skills are described as the child's **first messages**, and they provide an important and dynamic framework for the transition into being able to use first words and simple phrases.

First messages (also known as 'first meanings') and the approaches to developing them are described by Coupe O'Kane and Goldbart (1998), based on work by Bloom, Lahey and Leonard. Their significance in the development of communication skills came from the finding that 'many pupils were failing to develop functional communication at the single word level', and they believe this to be linked to the overemphasis on teaching vocabulary. Instead, the authors suggested that there should be a focus on extending the meanings and messages that the child conveys, and that this should at least lead to a more useful and better-used range of words or signs.

This 'First messages' section of this chapter therefore gives a structure and practical guide to identify the need and create the opportunity to communicate things that are most important from the child's point of view.

Routledge
Taylor & Francis Group
ROUTLEDGE

Communicative Intentions
why the child communicates

Communicative intentions describe the purpose or 'why' the child is communicating, and can be considered as forming the core communication framework into which the child's new skills gradually slot. For example, *how* a child requests a banana changes considerably:

* Crying and reaching towards a banana on the table
* Saying 'baba' whilst pointing at the banana
* Saying 'bana' to the adult
* 'Banana please'
* 'Can I have a banana please Mummy?'

But this linguistic-based development is secondary to the development of the child's skills in being able to make an 'I want …' request.

Another example of the reason why the child is communicating overriding the meaning of the actual word is illustrated by the way children first use the words 'Mummy' or 'Daddy' in order to get attention or help from anyone who will listen, rather than to refer to the person themselves – much to many parents' frustration.

The **later communicative intentions** section of this chapter provides us with an overview of more advanced uses of communication, and the section on **conversational skills** offers an overview of the higher level of communication skills which are essential in ensuring that a person is able to communicate effectively in a range of different situations.

Implications of this Framework

There are two important implications from the framework of what and why the child communicates. First, the most effective and natural approach to support the development of any child's communication development at this stage is to focus on expanding the messages, reasons and opportunities to communicate, rather than on the way the child is communicating them. Second is the importance of identifying those children who have specific difficulty in developing their use of communication.

Considering the communicative framework idea again; if the framework does not form, or there are gaps in its formation, then:

* The child will be restricted in the messages that he can communicate – often being replaced by behavioural meltdowns, which are stressful for everyone.

* A lot of the language skills that the child learns are unlikely to be used for any immediate communicative purpose. Some children can develop good technical language skills, being able to recite songs and use learnt phrases and dialogues from the television or video/DVDs, but are unable to use these same words or sentences to give you information or to ask for something that they want.
* And, of course, some children so dislike the social aspect of communicating that they only do so when the reason to communicate is for an essential or 'to die for' outcome.

There is therefore enormous value in revisiting these early intentions and making sure that the child has the skills to be able to communicate for these reasons, and that the environmental demands and the interaction style of the adults provide opportunities for the child to use them.

Finally, there are many children for whom communicating is so stressful that they will actively avoid it – supporting these children and their families needs a very sensitive balance between extending the child's communication skills and maintaining his 'comfort zone'.

Routledge
Taylor & Francis Group
ROUTLEDGE

Use of Communication Skills – Overview of Developmental Stages

Early Communicators	P-LEVEL
* SELF-INTERACTION	**P1(i) and P1(ii)**
* TWO-WAY INTERACTION	**P2(i)**
— With a person	
— With an object	
* THREE-WAY INTERACTION	**P2(ii)**
— Share joint attention	
— Follow joint attention	
* EARLY THREE-WAY COMMUNICATION	**P3(i)**
— Directs attention to self (starts an interaction)	
— Directs attention to get something (early 'I want that' request)	
— Directs attention to show something (early 'look at that' comment)	
Developing Communicators	
* ESTABLISHED THREE-WAY COMMUNICATION	**P3(ii)**
* FIRST MESSAGES	**P3(ii) – P5**
* EARLY COMMUNICATIVE INTENTIONS	**P3(ii) – P5**
Established Communicators	
* LATER COMMUNICATIVE INTENTIONS	**P6 – P8**
* CONVERSATIONAL SKILLS	**P6 – P8**

Each of these stages is explained in detail on pages 90–106.

Early Communicators

Involuntary reactions and reflexes

Adults instinctively respond to a child's state of comfort, distress, alertness and lack of interest, and from this interprets the following **meanings**:

* Like/want
* Dislike/reject

From the child's point of view his interaction focusses on experiencing and making sense of his internal states and his own involuntary actions, with little awareness of the outside world. This stage can therefore be referred to as one of '**self-interaction**'.

The adult focusses on building a relationship with the child through bursts of face-to-face play, with the purpose of creating a 'connection' and awareness between them. Typical games include the adult smiling, using exaggerated sounds, voices, movements and noises. Crucial to the adult carrying on with these games is that the child reacts, or is perceived to react, in some way; and this depends on the point at which the child develops an awareness of things in his environment that are external and separate from himself.

Some children with a learning disability will return to 'self interaction' as a predictable and safe experience, and sometimes as a way of self calming. Whilst some of these deliberate actions can be socially unacceptable and even cause the child harm – simply stopping them may cause the child enormous distress and, in my experience, bring about replacement with something worse.

Routledge P
Taylor & Francis Group
ROUTLEDGE

Voluntary reactions

Adults begin to see a pattern of different reactions to which they can attach the following **meanings**:

* Like
* Dislike
* Want
* Don't want

* Recognition
* Discomfort
* Interest
* Surprise

In addition, the adult begins to talk to the child about their interpretation of his behaviour. For example, the child smiles as he is being fed and the adult comments, 'Ooh, you like that don't you?', or the child turns to a voice, 'Oh, you know who your grandma is!'

The child's interaction focusses on the development of his ability to interact with things external to his own body: people and objects. However, during this stage, the child is only able to interact with one or the other, and cannot combine interacting with both at once. This can therefore be referred to as '**two-way interaction**' because it involves either the *child* interacting with an *object*, or the *child* interacting with an *adult*.

There are two stages of development:

* Initially, a rigid either/or interaction

The child is able to interact with things in his environment, but it is a rigid either/or focus; he can either play and interact with a person (commonly through face-to-face games and games on the adult's lap) or play with an object (usually through mouthing and holding) but not both at the same time.

For example, if an adult comes along whilst the child is looking at an object, the child will either ignore the adult and carry on, engrossed in his game, or, if the adult interrupts, the child will drop the object and focus entirely on the adult.

* Later, a flexible either/or interaction

Gradually, this shift in interaction focus becomes more flexible and the child appears to be able to maintain two parallel foci of attention. So if an adult comes along, the child looks up from his object and interacts briefly with the adult, for example smiles, and then the child goes back to his original activity of exploring his toy. Although the child does not drop one interaction in preference to the other, he still cannot combine his focus of interaction with both at once.

However, this incidental sequence, on the child's behalf, of looking up and then back to what he was doing, acts as a strong signal to the adult that the child is actually trying to engage them in his activity. The response of the adult to further comment and join in with the child's activity helps to shape the next stage of shared attention. (See page 92, 'If I do … I get …'.)

The combination of the child being able to use planned actions, together with his ability to anticipate what is about to happen within his routines, leads to more definite patterns of behaviour that make it far easier for adults to interpret the following **intents**:

* Like
* Dislike
* Want
* Don't want

* Discomfort
* Surprise
* Interest
* Recognition

The interaction changes from the simple adult–child interaction games, such as peek-a-boo, tickling, smiling and giggling, to the adult beginning to talk about and join in with his activities. For example:

* The adult interprets the child's actions: the child is playing with a toy and the adult comments, 'Oh you've got teddy, you like teddy, ahh ... cuddle teddy'
* The adult talks about what is happening in an activity: 'Here comes the spoon', 'Uh-oh, all fall down', 'Let's put on your shoes'
* The adult makes a comment about someone or something nearby, 'Look, there's Holly', 'Here's Mummy', 'Oh look at Verity, she's waving at you', and in this way draws the child's attention to it
* The adult interprets the child's 'reach-for-real' attempts as 'I want that', and responds by helping, making a comment and getting involved.

Through this process of the adult following the child's lead and joining in with whatever he is showing an interest in, the child begins to experience **'three-way interaction'**, that is, *the child* **combining his focus of interaction** with *an adult* and *an object (or event)*, at the same time.

There are two stages of development:

* Sharing joint attention

The adult creates the shared focus through commenting about and joining in with something the child is already looking at or playing with.

The child learns to share their focus of attention between an adult and object at the same time.

* Following joint attention

Gradually, within these shared games, the adult begins to direct the child's attention to something that he is not currently involved in at that moment, for example, to something nearby or to a different toy.

Routledge
Taylor & Francis Group
ROUTLEDGE

The child learns to respond to and follow the adult's focus of attention, by playing with the new toy (rather than sticking to the one he has already got), or looking in the direction to which the adult is pointing. Initially, this will be following a point to something the adult is touching, and then the distance gradually increases until the child is able to follow a point to something across the room or outside of the window. (Following a distance point may not be evident until P3(i), the next stage.)

The child now begins to direct his patterns of behaviours at the adult in order to deliberately involve them in doing things for him and with him; in this way the child begins to intentionally **communicate a message**.

However, these are only very emergent attempts, and the adults will still need to interpret a lot of the child's behaviours from the context, as before; but the key difference is that the child is now far more actively involved by initiating the message for himself, rather than the adults simply interpreting his response to something.

The most significant development within this stage is that the adult–child interaction changes from the child sharing and following the adult's focus of attention, to the child himself beginning to control and direct the adults focus of attention. It is this shift which enables the child to be able to direct his behaviours at the adult in order to communicate a message. This stage therefore marks the beginning of '**three-way communication**', that is, where *the child* **gains and directs a joint focus of attention** with *an adult* about *an object (or event)*. (See Appendices 4 and 5.)

There are two stages of development: first the child learns how to gain the adult's focus of attention and, second, how to direct it in order to get the desired response. However, these first attempts are rather muddled and it is often unclear whose attention the child is trying to gain and why. Within this stage, the child seems to focus his attention-gaining behaviours at *either* the adult *or* on the thing that he is trying to draw attention to, but he cannot coordinate both gaining and directing at once. This can therefore be called '**early three-way communication**'.

During this stage of early three-way communication the child uses these skills to:

* **Gain an adult's attention to himself** (which is also referred to as the skill of 'starting an interaction'). For example:
  — The child looks and smiles at an adult
  — He starts to make noises and body movements when an adult comes near

* **Direct the adult's attention to something that he wants** (forming an early 'I want that' request)

  This generally involves persistent attention-gaining behaviour directed either at the adult or towards the thing that the child wants, for example:
  — Making cross noises whilst looking at his cup as if it will, on its own, move off the table towards him
  — Or simply protesting to the adult – through any combination of noises and behaviours

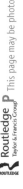

The adult may need to have a couple of guesses at what the child wants, but is left in no doubt that he wants something!

* **Direct an adult's attention to something nearby in order to show and share it** (forming an early 'look at this' comment)

  This generally involves the child directing his message at either the object or gaining the adult's attention, but not linking both:

  — The child points towards something or holds an object up, as if he is telling himself or the object something (as part of his own game)
  — Or he pulls the adult to somewhere but does not then direct them to what it is he wants the adult to look at or do

Again, it is the adult who needs to notice and interpret (or guess!) the child's behaviour. If they do not notice, the moment will be lost as the child does not direct the behaviour at anyone, nor does he persist in the behaviour.

Within this stage, 'If I do … You do …', there is a predominance of early three-way communication attempts changing to established three-way communication as the child moves towards the next stage of situational communication.

Developing Communicators

Early communicative intentions

Situational stage P3(ii)

The most important development within this stage is that the child begins to use **established three-way communication** skills, that is, the child is able to coordinate directing his communicative behaviours at both the adult (in order to gain their attention) and at an object/event (in order to direct the adult's attention to it), *at the same time*. (Two main reasons why the child wants to communicate then emerge: to request something and to tell you something.)

Examples

(i) To get something ('I want that' request):

The child uses attention-seeking behaviour directed at the adult and towards what he wants at the same time:

* Making a noise whilst looking at the adult (to gain the adult's attention) and then reaching and looking towards his cup (to direct the adult's attention), and repeating this is until the adult responds
* Rattling the cupboard door and screaming whilst also looking at the adult (to check that action is being taken!)
* Pulling the adult to the door and looking from the adult to the handle
* Or protesting loudly whilst pulling the adult towards something

The child is making it much more obvious what he wants the adult to do.

(ii) To show something ('Look at this' comment):

The child uses an object or a gesture to gain and direct the adult's attention so that they share the same focus of attention at the same time, ie creates *joint attention*:

* The child holds the toy up and looks towards the adult
* Or points towards something whilst looking at the adult
* Or he goes over and tugs the adult to something and then points

The child is now making it really clear what he wants the adult to pay attention to.

Overview of the early communicative intentions

Once the child's ability to use three-way communication is established these early requests and comments rapidly develop further, and the child's use of the early communicative intentions expands and develops across the whole of the Developing Communicators phase. There are initially many variations in the child's use of them,

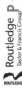

according to who the child is communicating with, the environment that he is in and

he wants to communicate about. However, as the child's skill in using them grows, he will be able to use a wider range of intentions, across a wider range of situations, and their use becomes more consistent and reliable.

Requesting

* Person (eg calls for Mummy)
* Object (eg tugs adult to cupboard, points to toy on shelf, says 'biscuit')
* Action or event (eg wants a cuddle, starts action-song, wants adult to put on a video, shouts at the back door to go in the garden)
* More (eg screams when you stop the game, tries to continue the same actions, wants more food or drink)
* Help (eg indicates that he needs help in opening lid on cup, or box of toys, rather than getting cross or abandoning his attempt)
* Information and asking questions (eg looks surprised when boots are not there and says 'boots?' with a questioning intonation)

Telling you something

* Naming (eg pictures, things around him)
* Making comments as events happen (eg saying 'hot' as he gets into the bath, or holding up his hands, saying 'sticky')
* Answering questions (eg pointing when asked, 'Where's your teddy?', or telling you where it is)
* Telling the adult about something that has happened (eg telling you 'Me falled over', or 'Dog ball mouth')

Rejecting

* Action or event (eg turns head away from approaching spoon)
* Object (eg pushes the offered toy away)
* Person (eg ignores all the adult's attempts to join in)

It is also essential to consider what role the child takes when communicating any of these intentions – is he:

* Initiating by starting the interaction himself (ie taking an **active role**)
* Responding when prompted (ie taking a **passive role**)

It is very important that the child has the opportunity to develop his skills in actively initiating interactions and, as a result, to experience other people responding to him. Ideally there should be a 50/50 balance between leading and responding, with neither person dominating.

REMEMBER: it is the reasons *why* the child is communicating rather than *how* he is communicating that is being looked at within this framework, so the examples are only to illustrate the points – there can be an enormous range of verbal and non-verbal behaviours used. In fact *how* the child communicates often stays the same and is intention-dependent (eg points for his teddy and screams for his cup) for some time whilst there is significant expansion in the reasons *why* the child uses his skills, which makes this 'use of communication' a more useful and relevant area in which to monitor the child's communicative progress.

For more detailed assessment, Coupe O'Kane and Goldbart (1998) and Dewart and Summers (1988) may be helpful.

There are two stages to the development of 'first messages':

First, the child recognises and understands what is going on:

* The biscuit tin is not in its usual place – the child may look around for it, he may walk away or he may get really cross with the cupboard; he knows that it should be there and it is not
* After Grandma has left the house and you have shut the door your child sits and waves to the door; he understands that someone has disappeared

This stage is often observed by the child using a range of behaviours which show that he understands what is going on, but does not try to tell anyone else about it. It is the equivalent of an 'early three-way communication', because it just involves the child directing his behaviours at the event.

Second, the child communicates about what the situation means to him:

* When he discovers that the biscuit tin is missing he pulls the adult to the cupboard or shouts for attention until they help
* As Grandma is leaving the house he begins to wave, communicating a 'bye' message

In this stage the child's behaviours are unmistakably directed at another person, making it 'established three-way communication', because the child is giving a message about the event to someone else.

First messages can be used to find out the range of things that the child communicates about and to plan natural, everyday situations to promote further development and use. The messages are generally communicated in a way which reflects the child's stage of expressive language development, that is, initially through behaviours (situational stage), then single words (first-words stage) and short phrases (simple phrases stage).

The following section outlines the messages and their meanings, and is illustrated by what the child might say if he had the words to do so.

Appeared (existence) *'I know what that is!', 'look at that!'*

The child communicates to:

* Tell you about things that they know and recognise
* Direct the adult's attention to something of interest and importance (to him)

For example, the child looks, points and vocalises/uses an early word at the dog or something he sees when he is out and about. Or he might hold something up towards the adult and say something. It might even be a related message, showing the child's understanding of a situation, for example saying 'quack quack' and pointing towards the park.

Disappeared (disappearance) *'all gone', 'bye bye'*

The child communicates to:

* Tell you about something that has disappeared, or is disappearing
* Request that something or someone disappears

For example, the child waves and says goodbye over your shoulder as you take him out of the room, waves goodbye to a person as he leaves the house, puts a toy into the bin saying, 'all gone', or simply hands over his cup to show you that his drink is finished. A favourite example of requesting something to disappear is my nephew bringing his Grandma's shoes over from the front door and then waving 'bye bye' to her when he wanted her to leave, and another child saying an agitated 'bye' to the new, and rather boisterous, puppy.

Stopped (recurrence) *'more', 'again', 'all gone', 'finished'*

The child communicates to:

* Tell you that something has stopped or ended
* Request for it to continue

For example, pulling the adult to the television to show that the DVD/video has stopped, bringing over a wind-up toy which has stopped moving, handing over his cup for another drink, or wanting another push on the swing or to be lifted back to the top of the slide (yet again!).

Gone missing (non-existence) *'gone', 'all gone …', '[name of thing]?' (with a questioning intonation), 'where's …?'*

The child communicates to:

* Tell you that something, or someone, is missing from its normal place
* Request information as to where it is (*asks a question*)

For example, the biscuit tin has not been put back in its usual place, or all the fruit has been eaten and the bowl is empty, or telling you that his sister is not at home – she has 'all gone'. At a later stage in the development it also includes the child using a simple question form to ask where the missing item is.

Routledge
Taylor & Francis Group
ROUTLEDGE

Where things are (location) *'there', '[name of place]', 'look', 'on', 'up'*

The child communicates to:

* Tell you where someone or something is
* Request that something or someone is put in that place
* Answer a 'where's …' question (*answers question*)

For example, telling you that the puppy is on the settee (again), spotting his favourite toy on the table and pointing at it delightedly, wanting to get up next to you or on you, or wanting to be put onto something (like the bed). Later in this stage of development it also includes responding to simple 'here and now' questions such as 'Where's Daddy?' with a point or words.

Whose is whose? (possession) *'mine'*

The child communicates to:

* Tell you about who owns what

For example, screaming when a sibling takes his cup or cake. Holding a jumper and saying, 'Daddy', or smiling when you hold his cup and say 'Whose is this?'

Rejection *'no way', 'stop', 'I do not want to do this', 'that's wrong'*

The child communicates to:

* Tell you that a person, object or event is not wanted
* Tell you when something is wrong
* Request that the current activity stops

Usually (and effectively) achieved by pushing things away, turning away, shaking the head, covering the mouth or eyes, or the use of a resounding 'No!' If the child has not developed a conventional way of communicating a rejection message, it is most commonly conveyed through a behavioural meltdown, which tends to intensify when things 'aren't right', particularly when the child's request has resulted in the wrong thing being given – for example, being given the 'wrong' juice (eg it's not apple).

To be in charge of something (be the activator) *'me', 'I want to do it', 'my turn', 'I want a go'*

The child communicates to:

* Request a go at something
* Request an object

For example, every time you try to feed the child with a spoon he turns his face away but then reaches for the spoon, or as you blow bubbles he grabs for the wand – he wants to do it for himself. Other examples include screaming when he sees a sibling playing with something that he wants (but inevitably cannot have), or shouting 'me, me, me' to get a turn at holding the rabbit or protesting in order to help stir the cake mixture.

To be on the receiving end of an action (be the receiver) *'and me', 'it is used for …', 'it is … turn'*

The child communicates to:

* Tell you about what things are associated with and used for
* Request that something happens to him or nominates someone else to be on the receiving end!

For example, the adult holds up a hairbrush and asks 'What is this?', and the child touches his hair to show what it should be used on; or a child brings a toothbrush over to the adult and puts it to his mouth. Other situations include: the child communicating that he wants to be included in an activity; for example, everyone is putting on their boots to go outside, or climbing into the car, and the child protests loudly that he does not want to be left out. Or requesting a particular action or event, for example, the child's sister get a tickle or a kiss and his Grandma is left in no doubt that he wants one too; or he tries to get the adult to sing a song, give him a cuddle or look at a book with him. This stage also includes the child making requests for something to happen to someone else; for example, when the teacher asks, 'Who wants a go?', the child nominates his friend rather than himself.

To comment on an activity (an action) *'up', 'go', 'uh-oh'*

The child communicates to:

* Tell you about mishaps: 'uh-oh' as he knocks over your drink or drops something off the table
* Tell you about what he is doing: 'go' as he rolls the ball, or 'up' as he is scrambling onto the bed

To comment on something (an attribute) *'yucky', 'nice', 'dirty'*

The child communicates to:

✳ Tell you about what he thinks of something

This results in some classic faces and reactions as the child tells you what he thinks about things — from your cooking to what he has found lurking under a stone!

Established Communicators

Later communicative intentions

These intentions are an extension to the core reasons to communicate, and they develop as the child acquires more sophisticated communication skills:

* Asks for confirmation of information ('Go dog walk?')
* Asks for clarification ('The red one?')
* Takes and gives messages ('Mummy says it's tidy-up time')
* Asks for help ('Help, help I stuck!')
* Directs others and gives instructions (tells another child when it is their turn, or what to do)
* Retells an event ('I got a cup drew round it and …')
* Describes ('I Florence', 'That's my Mummy!', 'That's really disgusting and yucky', 'A big green lorry')
* Talks about language using language (metalinguistic skills) ('Is it swimmed or swam?')
* Uses language to control a situation ('I haven't finished my turn yet')
* Pretends ('I'll be Mummy')
* Reasons, negotiates and bargains! ('What if …')
* Uses humour (wobbly jokes and dodgy playing on words)
* Talks about own feelings ('I've got an angry bug')
* Enquires about others' feelings ('You had a nice swim Daddy?')

The above only provides a summary overview of the skills involved in later communicative intentions, to enable discussion. For more detailed assessment and references see Anderson-Wood and Rae Smith (1997), Coupe O'Kane and Goldbart (1998), Dewart and Summers (1995) and Rinaldi (1992a).

Conversational skills

Conversations

∗ Gaining the listener's attention before starting to talk

∗ Starting up a conversation (*initiating*)

∗ Taking turns by:
— Taking a turn up
— Letting the other person in

∗ Keeping the conversation going (*maintaining*) by:
— Asking questions/answering questions
— Using statements/replying to statements

∗ Ending a conversation (*terminating*)

∗ Coping with misunderstandings (*repairing*) by:
— Recognising that a breakdown has occurred
— Getting the message across when the listener has not understood
— Asking for clarification when the child himself has not understood

∗ Showing that you are listening by:
— Looking at the speaker
— Making non-verbal responses (eg nods, facial expression)

∗ Managing topics of conversation by:
— Talking about the same thing as the other person or group
— Being able to change the topic appropriately

∗ Knowing when and how to interrupt

Body language

∗ Eye contact; this naturally varies:
— As the speaker
— As the listener

∗ Facial expression; appropriate facial expressions should reflect:
— The speaker's feelings
— The social context
— The content of message given or received

∗ Posture: this again should reflect the context and content of the conversation and also to be encouraging of having a conversation with that person in the first place.

∗ Fidgeting: a normal level of fidgeting is needed to keep alert and to concentrate; however, it is inappropriate if it gets to the level where it distracts the conversational partner.

* Distance from the person you are talking to: this should not be too close (or too far), and touching should be appropriate to the context and to the relationship between the speaker and listener

How you talk

If any one of the following skills is impaired, it will affect the child's conversational style and, most significantly, the way that people respond to him:

* Volume
* Tone
* Speed
* Intelligibility
* Fluency

Awareness of the listener's needs (presupposition)

This involves looking at how good the child is at seeing the conversation from the listener's point of view, and adjusting his style and the content accordingly. This includes:

* Talking about things in the right amount of detail – taking account of what the listener already knows or needs to know

* Clearly establishing who and what he is talking about, and the timescale, which involves the appropriate use of referents in order to avoid sentences like 'Then he went there'

* Using the right style of communication and vocabulary for the situation, that is, adapting the style and content to the listener's mood, level of interest and relationship to the child

* Being generally relevant

The above only provides a summary overview of the skills involved in conversational skills, to enable discussion and identification of the key areas that need further investigation or support. For more detailed assessment and references see Kelly (1996) and Rinaldi (1992a, 1992b).

Routledge
Taylor & Francis Group
ROUTLEDGE

This page may be photocopied for instructional use only. *The Communication Development Profile* © Charlotte Child 2006

Appendices

Appendix 1 How the Child's Understanding of Spoken Language Develops

Children begin to respond to what you say when they understand what you mean. At this stage their understanding of what you mean does not come from the words that you say, but from:

* Your actions
* Your tone of voice and body language
* The child's familiarity with what is going on, and with what is usually expected of him in that situation

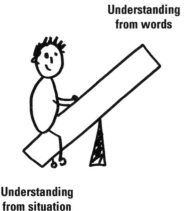

Fig 1 *Child understands from the situation rather than from words.*

Understanding from words

Understanding from situation

> The child uses the situation to work out what is being said – so what you are doing is far more important than what you are saying.

Gradually, this reliance shifts, like a see-saw, as the child begins to understand:

* Naming words   * Action words

He can pick up and respond to one or two of these words in a sentence. The child continues to rely on working out the rest of the meaning from interpreting what is going on around him.

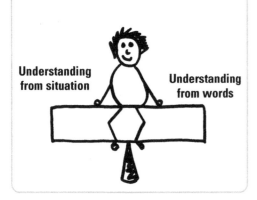

Fig 2 *Child understands equally from the situation and from what is being said*

Understanding from situation

Understanding from words

> The situation and the words are equally important for the child to be able to work out the meaning of what is being said.

Finally, the child develops his understanding of:

* Describing words   * Grammatical information

He can pick up and respond to three or four words in a sentence. As a result, the child is able to understand most of what has been said from the words alone.

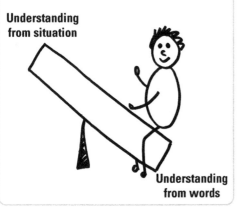

Fig 3 *Child is able to understand what has been said from words alone*

Understanding from situation

Understanding from words

> The child has an independent understanding of spoken language.

However, the child needs to continue to use a certain amount of situational information to help him to work out any additional meaning over and above the words; this is conveyed through, for example, the use of sarcasm, tone of voice, inference, facial expressions and body language etc. Where this skill does not develop, the child is at risk of making 'literal interpretations'.

Routledge
Taylor & Francis Group
ROUTLEDGE

Naming Words

Action Words

Describing Words

Grammar

This maps onto Appendix 3

Routledge
Taylor & Francis Group
ROUTLEDGE

One Word

Two Words

Three Words

Four Words

Routledge
Taylor & Francis Group
ROUTLEDGE

Routledge
Taylor & Francis Group
ROUTLEDGE

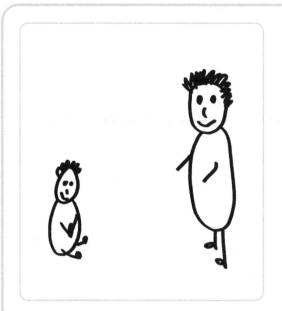

1 Share joint attention

Fig 4 *Child playing, adult joins in*

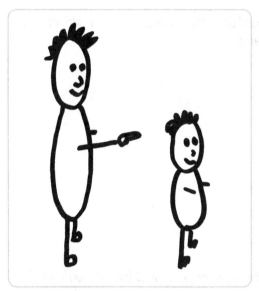

2 Follow joint attention

Fig 5 *Adult directs, child responds.*

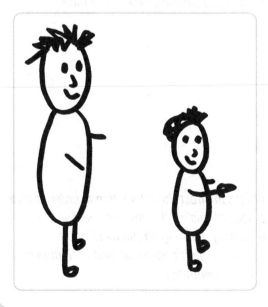

3 Direct joint attention

Fig 6 *Child directs, adult responds*

Appendix 5   How Three-Way Communication Develops

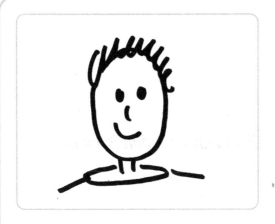

1 Self-interaction

Fig 7   *Child focussed on his own body feedback*

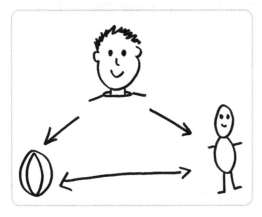

2 Two-way interactions

Fig 8   *Child can interact with either an object or a person*

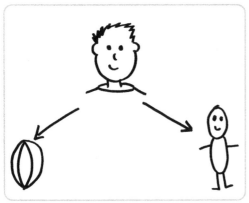

3 Three-way interactions

Fig 9   *Child can focus on, and interact with, an object and a person at the same time.*

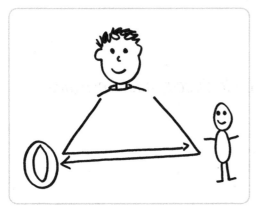

4 Three-way communication

Fig 10   *Child can direct the interaction in order to give a 'look at this' or 'I want this' message by:*
– holding up/bringing things to adult
– gaining adult's attention and then directing it to something.

Routledge
Taylor & Francis Group
ROUTLEDGE

Case Study

The Communication Development Profile can be used across a whole range of environments but this case study is a typical example of how the profile supports children with special needs in a mainstream school setting. The names of teacher, parent and child have been changed.

Peter is 7 years old and attends his local primary school. He has severe learning difficulties and has a full time learning support assistant. His teacher reports that he does not communicate much in class and that she is finding it really hard to set new targets, or more importantly, targets that make a difference to the way that he interacts and communicates with everyone. His parents are very supportive but are concerned that he is not being seen in the best light, and they report that at home he uses lots of words, even sentences, and has no difficulty in understanding what has been said.

Stage 1

A formal assessment and observation by me quickly indicated that Peter was around the two-word level for both his comprehension and expression. It was clear that his one-word level skills were the most consistent but he was beginning to achieve some early two-word level skills.

He could listen and follow adult directions for a task providing the adult gained and maintained his attention throughout, and his sound system was developing in line with his language skills.

Stage 2

The next stage was to meet Peter's parents and his teaching team. At this meeting we used the Communication Development Profile to discuss and agree how Peter's communication skills were developing and to identify how we could best help and support him.

This was achieved by looking at the descriptions for each communication skill at the level I felt Peter was at from the formal assessment and observation. His parents and teacher then used this to discuss their experiences of Peter's communication skills. By looking at what would be expected of a child at the stage above as well as the stage below we were able to agree each level.

The 'Use of communication skills' section ('What and why the child communicates') was completed through joint discussion, and from it everyone became more aware that although Peter did have a lot of words and signs that he could use, he often did not need to, or he was prompted to do so. We then agreed to focus on expanding his use of messages within school and at home, and targets were set to encourage this.

The following screens show how the Communication Development Profile questionnaires were used to build Peter's profile.

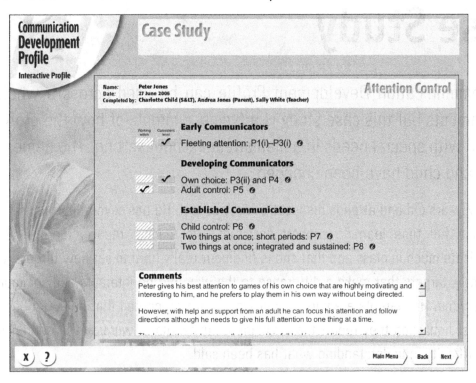

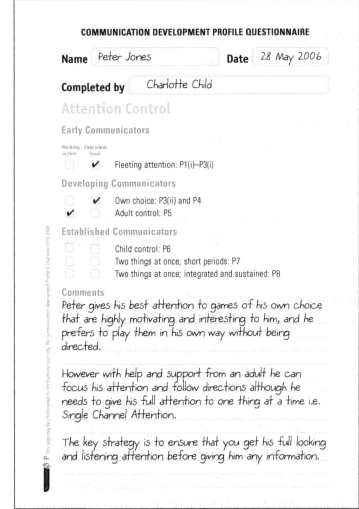

COMMUNICATION DEVELOPMENT PROFILE QUESTIONNAIRE

Name Peter Jones   Date 28 May 2006

Completed by   Charlotte Child

Attention Control

Early Communicators

Working within / Consistent level

☐ ✔ Fleeting attention: P1(i)–P3(i)

Developing Communicators

☐ ✔ Own choice: P3(ii) and P4
✔ ☐ Adult control: P5

Established Communicators

☐ ☐ Child control: P6
☐ ☐ Two things at once; short periods: P7
☐ ☐ Two things at once; integrated and sustained: P8

Comments

Peter gives his best attention to games of his own choice that are highly motivating and interesting to him, and he prefers to play them in his own way without being directed.

However with help and support from an adult he can focus his attention and follow directions although he needs to give his full attention to one thing at a time i.e. Single Channel Attention.

The key strategy is to ensure that you get his full looking and listening attention before giving him any information.

COMMUNICATION DEVELOPMENT PROFILE QUESTIONNAIRE

Name Peter Jones   Date 28 May 2006

Completed by   Charlotte Child

Continuation Sheet

(Copy this sheet as many times as you need)

How to help
1. start sentences with his name: 'Peter ...'
2. use 'Peter listen' to focus his attention.
3. remove anything that he can fiddle with, so that he focuses only on what you are saying.
4. try to be at his physical level, preferably facing him, so that you are making it really clear you are talking to him. Speaking to him from behind, across a room or even to the side can be less effective.

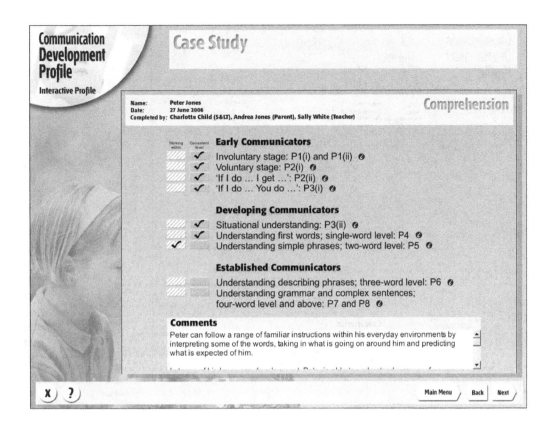

Communication Development Profile
Interactive Profile

Case Study

Name: **Peter Jones**
Date: **27 June 2006**
Completed by: **Charlotte Child (S&LT), Andrea Jones (Parent), Sally White (Teacher)**

Comprehension

Working within	Consistent level	
	✔	**Early Communicators**
	✔	Involuntary stage: P1(i) and P1(ii)
	✔	Voluntary stage: P2(i)
	✔	'If I do ... I get ...': P2(ii)
	✔	'If I do ... You do ...': P3(i)

Developing Communicators
Situational understanding: P3(ii)
Understanding first words; single-word level: P4
Understanding simple phrases; two-word level: P5

Established Communicators
Understanding describing phrases; three-word level: P6
Understanding grammar and complex sentences;
four-word level and above: P7 and P8

Comments
Peter can follow a range of familiar instructions within his everyday environments by interpreting some of the words, taking in what is going on around him and predicting what is expected of him.

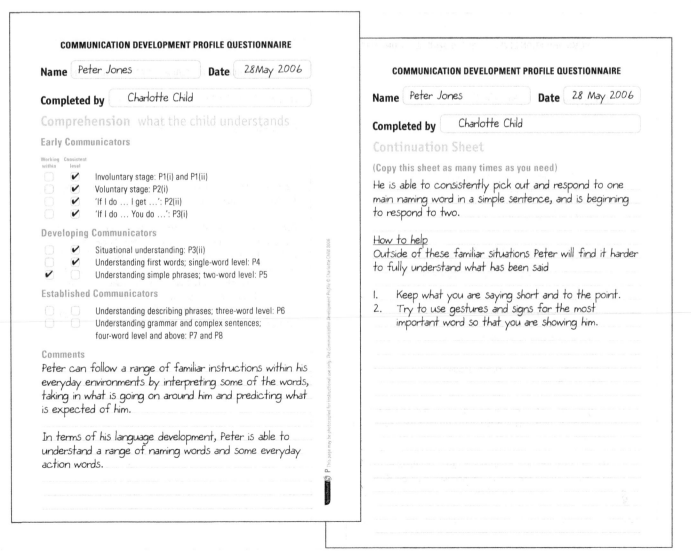

COMMUNICATION DEVELOPMENT PROFILE QUESTIONNAIRE

Name Peter Jones   **Date** 28 May 2006

Completed by Charlotte Child

Comprehension what the child understands

Early Communicators

Working within	Consistent level	
☐	✔	Involuntary stage: P1(i) and P1(ii)
☐	✔	Voluntary stage: P2(i)
☐	✔	'If I do ... I get ...': P2(ii)
☐	✔	'If I do ... You do ...': P3(i)

Developing Communicators

☐	✔	Situational understanding: P3(ii)
☐	✔	Understanding first words; single-word level: P4
✔	☐	Understanding simple phrases; two-word level: P5

Established Communicators

☐	☐	Understanding describing phrases; three-word level: P6
☐	☐	Understanding grammar and complex sentences; four-word level and above: P7 and P8

Comments
Peter can follow a range of familiar instructions within his everyday environments by interpreting some of the words, taking in what is going on around him and predicting what is expected of him.

In terms of his language development, Peter is able to understand a range of naming words and some everyday action words.

COMMUNICATION DEVELOPMENT PROFILE QUESTIONNAIRE

Name Peter Jones   **Date** 28 May 2006

Completed by Charlotte Child

Continuation Sheet

(Copy this sheet as many times as you need)

He is able to consistently pick out and respond to one main naming word in a simple sentence, and is beginning to respond to two.

How to help
Outside of these familiar situations Peter will find it harder to fully understand what has been said

1. Keep what you are saying short and to the point.
2. Try to use gestures and signs for the most important word so that you are showing him.

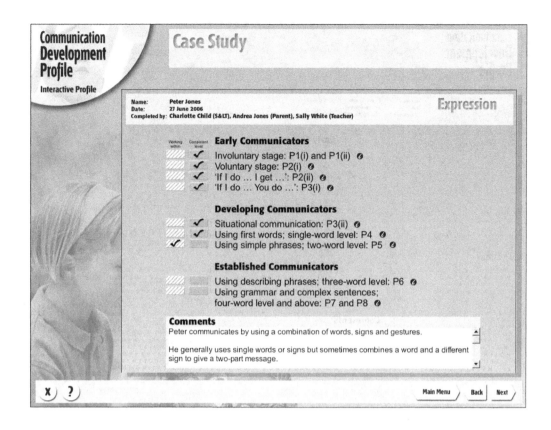

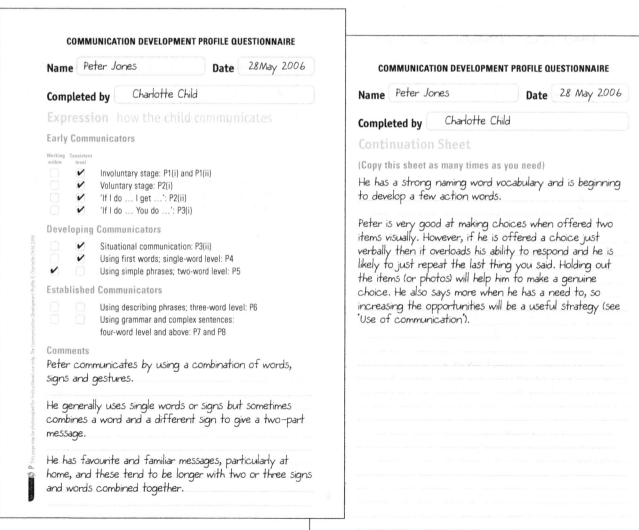

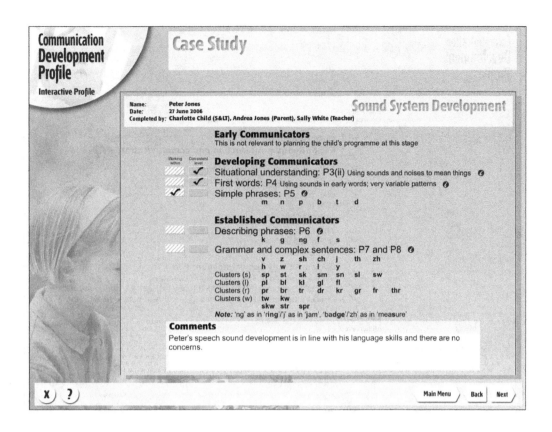

COMMUNICATION DEVELOPMENT PROFILE QUESTIONNAIRE

Name Peter Jones   **Date** 28 May 2006

Completed by   Charlotte Child

Sound System Development

Early Communicators

This is not relevant to planning the child's programme at this stage

Developing Communicators

Working within	Consistent level	
☐	✔	Situational understanding: P3(ii)
		Using sounds and noises to mean things
☐	✔	First words: P4
		Using sounds in early words; very variable patterns
✔	☐	Simple phrases: P5
		m n p b t d

Established Communicators

☐	☐	Describing phrases: P6
		k g ng f s
☐	☐	Grammar and complex sentences: P7 and P8
		v z sh ch j th zh
		h w r l y

Clusters (s) sp st sk sm sn sl sw
Clusters (l)   pl bl kl gl fl
Clusters (r) pr br tr dr kr gr fr thr
Clusters (w) tw kw
           skw str spr

Note: 'ng' as in 'ri**ng**'/'j' as in '**j**am', 'ba**dge**'/'zh' as in 'mea**s**ure'

Comments

Peter's speech sound development is in line with his language skills and there are no concerns.

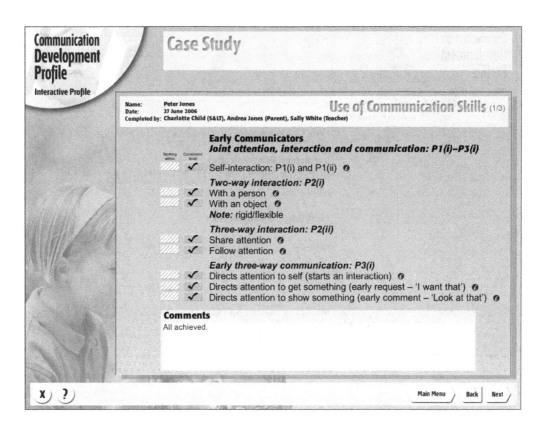

Case Study

Name: Peter Jones
Date: 27 June 2006
Completed by: Charlotte Child (S&LT), Andrea Jones (Parent), Sally White (Teacher)

Use of Communication Skills (1/3)

Early Communicators
Joint attention, interaction and communication: P1(i)–P3(i)

Working within / Consistent level

✓ Self-interaction: P1(i) and P1(ii)

Two-way interaction: P2(i)
✓ With a person
✓ With an object
Note: rigid/flexible

Three-way interaction: P2(ii)
✓ Share attention
✓ Follow attention

Early three-way communication: P3(i)
✓ Directs attention to self (starts an interaction)
✓ Directs attention to get something (early request – 'I want that')
✓ Directs attention to show something (early comment – 'Look at that')

Comments
All achieved.

Main Menu ⟩ Back Next ⟩

COMMUNICATION DEVELOPMENT PROFILE QUESTIONNAIRE

Name Peter Jones   **Date** 28 May 2006

Completed by Charlotte Child

Use of Communication Skills
what and why the child communicates

Early Communicators

Joint attention, interaction and communication: P1(i)–P3(i)

Working within / Consistent level

✔ *Self-interaction:* P1(i) and P1(ii)

Two-way interaction: P2(i)
✔ With a person
✔ With an object
Note: rigid/flexible

Three-way interaction: P2(ii)
✔ Share attention
✔ Follow attention

Early three-way communication: P3(i)
✔ Directs attention to self (*starts an interaction*)
✔ Directs attention to get something (*early request – 'I want that'*)
✔ Directs attention to show something (*early comment – 'Look at that'*)

Comments
All achieved.

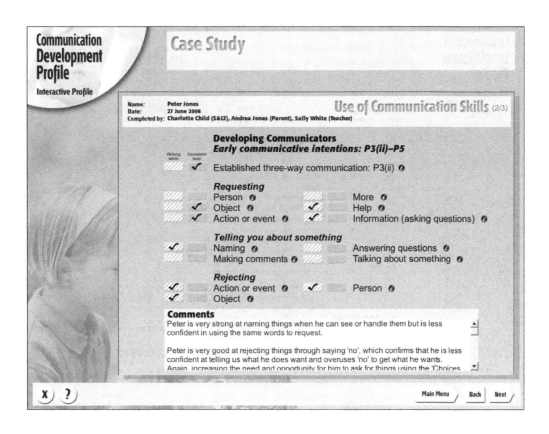

Communication Development Profile
Interactive Profile

Case Study

Name: **Peter Jones**
Date: **27 June 2006**
Completed by: **Charlotte Child (S&LT), Andrea Jones (Parent), Sally White (Teacher)**

Use of Communication Skills (2/3)

Developing Communicators
Early communicative intentions: P3(ii)–P5

Working within | Consistent level
✓ Established three-way communication: P3(ii) ⊘

Requesting
Person ⊘ — More ⊘
✓ Object ⊘ — ✓ Help ⊘
✓ Action or event ⊘ — ✓ Information (asking questions) ⊘

Telling you about something
✓ Naming ⊘ — Answering questions ⊘
Making comments ⊘ — Talking about something ⊘

Rejecting
✓ Action or event ⊘ — ✓ Person ⊘
✓ Object ⊘

Comments
Peter is very strong at naming things when he can see or handle them but is less confident in using the same words to request.

Peter is very good at rejecting things through saying 'no', which confirms that he is less confident at telling us what he does want and overuses 'no' to get what he wants. Again, increasing the need and opportunity for him to ask for things using the 'Choices

X ? | Main Menu › Back | Next ›

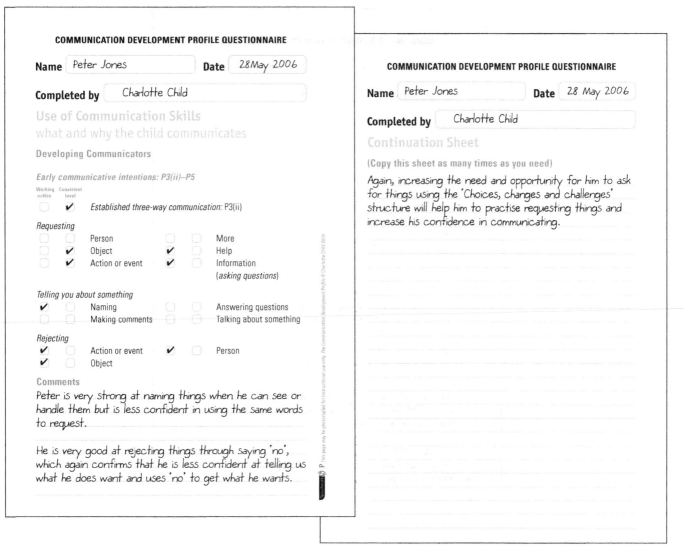

COMMUNICATION DEVELOPMENT PROFILE QUESTIONNAIRE

Name Peter Jones **Date** 28 May 2006

Completed by Charlotte Child

Use of Communication Skills
what and why the child communicates

Developing Communicators

Early communicative intentions: P3(ii)–P5

Working within | Consistent level
☐ ✓ *Established three-way communication:* P3(ii)

Requesting
☐ ☐ Person — ☐ ☐ More
☐ ✔ Object — ✔ ☐ Help
☐ ✔ Action or event — ✔ ☐ Information
(*asking questions*)

Telling you about something
✔ ☐ Naming — ☐ ☐ Answering questions
☐ ☐ Making comments — ☐ ☐ Talking about something

Rejecting
✔ ☐ Action or event — ✔ ☐ Person
✔ ☐ Object

Comments

Peter is very strong at naming things when he can see or handle them but is less confident in using the same words to request.

He is very good at rejecting things through saying 'no', which again confirms that he is less confident at telling us what he does want and uses 'no' to get what he wants.

COMMUNICATION DEVELOPMENT PROFILE QUESTIONNAIRE

Name Peter Jones **Date** 28 May 2006

Completed by Charlotte Child

Continuation Sheet

(Copy this sheet as many times as you need)

Again, increasing the need and opportunity for him to ask for things using the 'Choices, changes and challenges' structure will help him to practise requesting things and increase his confidence in communicating.

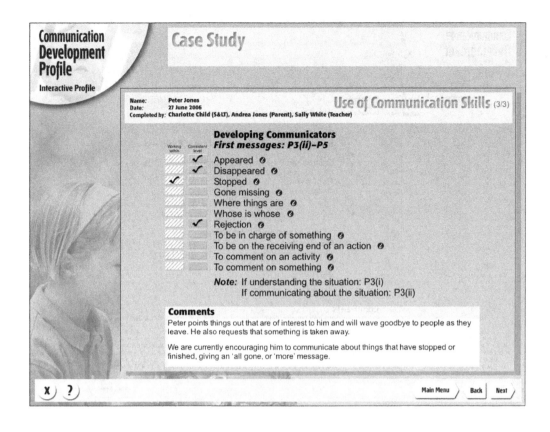

Communication Development Profile

Interactive Profile

Case Study

Name: Peter Jones
Date: 27 June 2006
Completed by: Charlotte Child (S&LT), Andrea Jones (Parent), Sally White (Teacher)

Use of Communication Skills (3/3)

Developing Communicators
First messages: P3(ii)–P5

Working within	Consistent level	
	✓	Appeared
	✓	Disappeared
✓		Stopped
		Gone missing
		Where things are
		Whose is whose
	✓	Rejection
		To be in charge of something
		To be on the receiving end of an action
		To comment on an activity
		To comment on something

Note: If understanding the situation: P3(i)
If communicating about the situation: P3(ii)

Comments
Peter points things out that are of interest to him and will wave goodbye to people as they leave. He also requests that something is taken away.

We are currently encouraging him to communicate about things that have stopped or finished, giving an 'all gone, or 'more' message.

X   ?   Main Menu   Back   Next

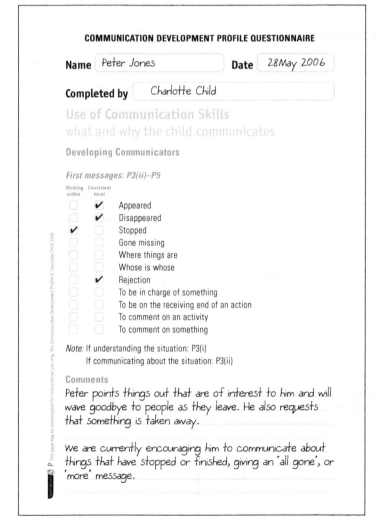

COMMUNICATION DEVELOPMENT PROFILE QUESTIONNAIRE

Name Peter Jones   **Date** 28May 2006

Completed by Charlotte Child

Use of Communication Skills
what and why the child communicates

Developing Communicators

First messages: P3(ii)–P5

Working within	Consistent level	
	✔	Appeared
	✔	Disappeared
✔		Stopped
		Gone missing
		Where things are
		Whose is whose
	✔	Rejection
		To be in charge of something
		To be on the receiving end of an action
		To comment on an activity
		To comment on something

Note: If understanding the situation: P3(i)
If communicating about the situation: P3(ii)

Comments
Peter points things out that are of interest to him and will wave goodbye to people as they leave. He also requests that something is taken away.

We are currently encouraging him to communicate about things that have stopped or finished, giving an 'all gone', or 'more' message.

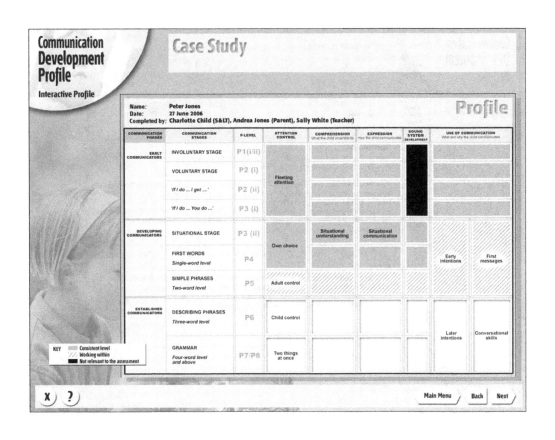

COMMUNICATION DEVELOPMENT PROFILE GRID

Name Peter Jones   **Date** 28 May 2006   **Completed by** Charlotte Child

COMMUNICATION PHASES	COMMUNICATION STAGES	P-LEVEL	ATTENTION CONTROL	COMPREHENSION *What the child understands*	EXPRESSION *How the child communicates*	SOUND SYSTEM	USE OF COMMUNICATION *What and why the child communicates*	
EARLY COMMUNICATORS	INVOLUNTARY STAGE	P1(i/ii)	Fleeting attention					
	VOLUNTARY STAGE	P2(i)						
	'If I do ... I get ...'	P2(ii)						
	'If I do ... You do ...'	P3(i)						
DEVELOPING COMMUNICATORS	SITUATIONAL STAGE	P3(ii)	Own choice	Situational understanding	Situational communication			
	FIRST WORDS *Single-word level*	P4					Early intentions	First messages
	SIMPLE PHRASES *Two-word level*	P5	Adult control					
ESTABLISHED COMMUNICATORS	DESCRIBING PHRASES *Three-word level*	P6	Child control				Later intentions	Conversational skills
	GRAMMAR *Four-word level and above*	P7/P8	Two things at once					

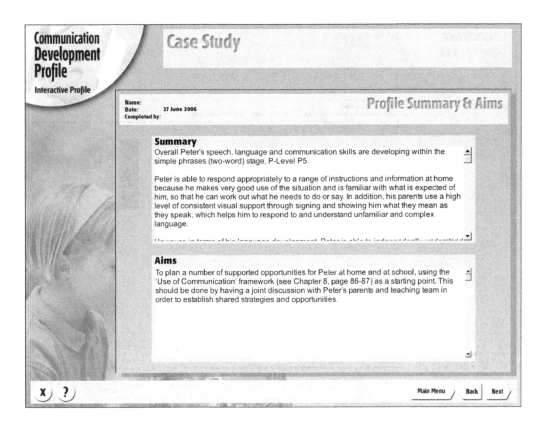

Case Study

Communication Development Profile
Interactive Profile

Name:
Date: 27 June 2006
Completed by:

Profile Summary & Aims

Summary

Overall Peter's speech, language and communication skills are developing within the simple phrases (two-word) stage, P-Level P5.

Peter is able to respond appropriately to a range of instructions and information at home because he makes very good use of the situation and is familiar with what is expected of him, so that he can work out what he needs to do or say. In addition, his parents use a high level of consistent visual support through signing and showing him what they mean as they speak, which helps him to respond to and understand unfamiliar and complex language.

Aims

To plan a number of supported opportunities for Peter at home and at school, using the 'Use of Communication' framework (see Chapter 8, page 86-87) as a starting point. This should be done by having a joint discussion with Peter's parents and teaching team in order to establish shared strategies and opportunities.

Main Menu   Back   Next

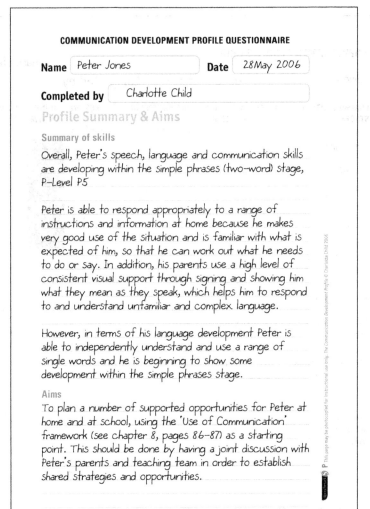

COMMUNICATION DEVELOPMENT PROFILE QUESTIONNAIRE

Name Peter Jones   **Date** 28 May 2006

Completed by Charlotte Child

Profile Summary & Aims

Summary of skills

Overall, Peter's speech, language and communication skills are developing within the simple phrases (two-word) stage, P-Level P5

Peter is able to respond appropriately to a range of instructions and information at home because he makes very good use of the situation and is familiar with what is expected of him, so that he can work out what he needs to do or say. In addition, his parents use a high level of consistent visual support through signing and showing him what they mean as they speak, which helps him to respond to and understand unfamiliar and complex language.

However, in terms of his language development Peter is able to independently understand and use a range of single words and he is beginning to show some development within the simple phrases stage.

Aims

To plan a number of supported opportunities for Peter at home and at school, using the 'Use of Communication' framework (see chapter 8, pages 86-87) as a starting point. This should be done by having a joint discussion with Peter's parents and teaching team in order to establish shared strategies and opportunities.

Peter's Profile

From the completed profile it is evident that Peter's overall stage of development falls within the Developing Communicators phase. He therefore needs to further develop his communication skills through closely matched and responsive everyday interactions, and not through a table top teaching approach. The aims and strategies to achieve these targets were then discussed together and it was agreed that the speech & language therapist would review their progress in six weeks but could be contacted by phone if there were any concerns in the meantime.

The Profile was used by me to have a joint discussion with Peter's parents and teaching team. This benefited both parties in several ways:

* the teaching team and parents both gained a better understanding of how communication skills develop, and what to look for.

* Peter's parents recognised how much he used his daily routine and visual clues to work out what was being said to him, and better understood his developing level of comprehension when he didn't have that same level of support.

* Peter's parents also realised the difference between using a series of individual words and putting words together to make a sentence, and we all reached agreement that Peter uses mostly single words and some combinations of a word plus a sign.

* In addition it became clear that Peter needed lots of prompts to use his words at home, and we were able to discuss moving on from this.

* Peter's teaching team recognised how few opportunities they were offering Peter to be able to communicate in class. Most things were anticipated and supplied and it was easy for Peter to 'go with the flow'. The messages section offered them a natural 'everyday' way of encouraging him to communicate with his teachers and friends in class.

Photocopiable Blank Profile Grid & Questionnaires

Communication Development Profile grid

Attention Control

Comprehension: what the child understands

Expression: how the child communicates

Sound System Development

Use of Communication Skills: what and why the child communicates

Summary & aims

The following pages contain the Profile Grid and Questionnaires that make up the Communication Development Profile. They can also be found on the CD-ROM.

Routledge
Taylor & Francis Group
ROUTLEDGE

COMMUNICATION DEVELOPMENT PROFILE GRID

Name [ ] Date [ ] Completed by [ ]

COMMUNICATION PHASES	COMMUNICATION STAGES	P-LEVEL	ATTENTION CONTROL	COMPREHENSION *What the child understands*	EXPRESSION *How child communicates*	SOUND SYSTEM	USE OF COMMUNICATION *What and why the child communicates*
EARLY COMMUNICATORS	INVOLUNTARY STAGE	P1(i/ii)					
	VOLUNTARY STAGE	P2(i)					
	'If I do … I get …'	P2(ii)	Fleeting attention				
	'If I do … You do …'	P3(i)					
DEVELOPING COMMUNICATORS	SITUATIONAL STAGE	P3(ii)		Situational understanding	Situational communication		Early intentions / First messages
	FIRST WORDS *Single-word level*	P4	Own choice				
	SIMPLE PHRASES *Two-word level*	P5	Adult control				
ESTABLISHED COMMUNICATORS	DESCRIBING PHRASES *Three-word level*	P6	Child control				Later intentions / Conversational skills
	GRAMMAR *Four-word level and above*	P7/P8	Two things at once				

Legend: ■ Area not relevant to the assessment ▢ Consistent level ▨ Working within

Routledge P Taylor & Francis Group This page may be photocopied for instructional use only. *The Communication Development Profile* © Charlotte Child 2006

COMMUNICATION DEVELOPMENT PROFILE QUESTIONNAIRE

Name [   ]   **Date** [   ]

Completed by [   ]

Attention Control

Early Communicators

Working within	Consistent level
☐	☐ Fleeting attention: P1(i)–P3(i)

Developing Communicators

☐ ☐ Own choice: P3(ii) and P4
☐ ☐ Adult control: P5

Established Communicators

☐ ☐ Child control: P6
☐ ☐ Two things at once; short periods: P7
☐ ☐ Two things at once; integrated and sustained: P8

Comments

_____

_____

_____

_____

_____

_____

_____

_____

_____

_____

_____

_____

_____

COMMUNICATION DEVELOPMENT PROFILE QUESTIONNAIRE

Name [ ] **Date** [ ]

Completed by [ ]

Comprehension what the child understands

Early Communicators

Working within	Consistent level	
☐	☐	Involuntary stage: P1(i) and P1(ii)
☐	☐	Voluntary stage: P2(i)
☐	☐	'If I do … I get …': P2(ii)
☐	☐	'If I do … You do …': P3(i)

Developing Communicators

☐	☐	Situational understanding: P3(ii)
☐	☐	Understanding first words; single-word level: P4
☐	☐	Understanding simple phrases; two-word level: P5

Established Communicators

☐	☐	Understanding describing phrases; three-word level: P6
☐	☐	Understanding grammar and complex sentences; four-word level and above: P7 and P8

Comments

_____

_____

_____

_____

_____

_____

_____

_____

_____

Routledge Taylor & Francis Group ROUTLEDGE

COMMUNICATION DEVELOPMENT PROFILE QUESTIONNAIRE

Name [   ]   **Date** [   ]

Completed by [   ]

Expression how the child communicates

Early Communicators

Working within	Consistent level	
☐	☐	Involuntary stage: P1(i) and P1(ii)
☐	☐	Voluntary stage: P2(i)
☐	☐	'If I do ... I get ...': P2(ii)
☐	☐	'If I do ... You do ...': P3(i)

Developing Communicators

☐	☐	Situational communication: P3(ii)
☐	☐	Using first words; single-word level: P4
☐	☐	Using simple phrases; two-word level: P5

Established Communicators

☐	☐	Using describing phrases; three-word level: P6
☐	☐	Using grammar and complex sentences: four-word level and above: P7 and P8

Comments

_____

_____

_____

_____

_____

_____

_____

_____

_____

Routledge
Taylor & Francis Group
ROUTLEDGE

COMMUNICATION DEVELOPMENT PROFILE QUESTIONNAIRE

Name [ ]   **Date** [ ]

Completed by [ ]

Sound System Development

Early Communicators

This is not relevant to planning the child's programme at this stage

Developing Communicators

Working within	Consistent level	
☐	☐	Situational understanding: P3(ii)
		Using sounds and noises to mean things
☐	☐	First words: P4
		Using sounds in early words; very variable patterns
☐	☐	Simple phrases: P5

m   n   p   b   t   d

Established Communicators

Working within	Consistent level	
☐	☐	Describing phrases: P6

k   g   ng   f   s

☐	☐	Grammar and complex sentences: P7 and P8

v   z   sh   ch   j   th   zh

h   w   r   l   y

Clusters (s)	sp	st	sk	sm	sn	sl	sw
Clusters (l)	pl	bl	kl	gl	fl
Clusters (r)	pr	br	tr	dr	kr	gr	fr	thr
Clusters (w)	tw	kw
	skw	str	spr

Note: 'ng' as in 'ri**ng**'/'j' as in '**j**am', 'ba**dge**'/'zh' as in 'mea**s**ure'

Comments

_____

_____

_____

COMMUNICATION DEVELOPMENT PROFILE QUESTIONNAIRE

Name [   ]   **Date** [   ]

Completed by [   ]

Use of Communication Skills
what and why the child communicates

Early Communicators

Joint attention, interaction and communication: P1(i)–P3(i)

Working within	Consistent level
☐	☐	*Self-interaction:* P1(i) and P1(ii)

Two-way interaction: P2(i)

Working within | Consistent level |
:---:|:---:|---
☐ | ☐ | With a person
☐ | ☐ | With an object
| | *Note:* rigid/flexible

Three-way interaction: P2(ii)

Working within | Consistent level |
:---:|:---:|---
☐ | ☐ | Share attention
☐ | ☐ | Follow attention

Early three-way communication: P3(i)

Working within | Consistent level |
:---:|:---:|---
☐ | ☐ | Directs attention to self (*starts an interaction*)
☐ | ☐ | Directs attention to get something (*early request – 'I want that'*)
☐ | ☐ | Directs attention to show something (*early comment – 'Look at that'*)

Comments

_____

_____

_____

_____

_____

_____

COMMUNICATION DEVELOPMENT PROFILE QUESTIONNAIRE

Name ☐   **Date** ☐

Completed by ☐

Use of Communication Skills
what and why the child communicates

Developing Communicators

Early communicative intentions: P3(ii)–P5

Working within	Consistent level		
☐	☐	*Established three-way communication: P3(ii)*	

Requesting

☐	☐	Person	☐	☐	More
☐	☐	Object	☐	☐	Help
☐	☐	Action or event	☐	☐	Information (*asking questions*)

Telling you about something

☐	☐	Naming	☐	☐	Answering questions
☐	☐	Making comments	☐	☐	Talking about something

Rejecting

☐	☐	Action or event	☐	☐	Person
☐	☐	Object			

Comments

_____

_____

_____

_____

_____

_____

_____

COMMUNICATION DEVELOPMENT PROFILE QUESTIONNAIRE

Name [   ] **Date** [   ]

Completed by [   ]

Use of Communication Skills
what and why the child communicates

Developing Communicators

First messages: P3(ii)–P5

Working within	Consistent level	
☐	☐	Appeared
☐	☐	Disappeared
☐	☐	Stopped
☐	☐	Gone missing
☐	☐	Where things are
☐	☐	Whose is whose
☐	☐	Rejection
☐	☐	To be in charge of something
☐	☐	To be on the receiving end of an action
☐	☐	To comment on an activity
☐	☐	To comment on something

Note: If understanding the situation: P3(i)

If communicating about the situation: P3(ii)

Comments

_____

_____

_____

_____

_____

_____

_____

Routledge
Taylor & Francis Group
ROUTLEDGE

COMMUNICATION DEVELOPMENT PROFILE QUESTIONNAIRE

Name [   ] **Date** [   ]

Completed by [   ]

Use of Communication Skills
what and why the child communicates

Established Communicators

Later communicative intentions: P6–P8

Working within	Consistent level	
☐	☐	Asks for confirmation of information
☐	☐	Asks for clarification
☐	☐	Takes and gives messages
☐	☐	Asks for help
☐	☐	Directs others and gives instructions
☐	☐	Retells an event
☐	☐	Describes
☐	☐	Talks about language using language
☐	☐	Uses language to control a situation
☐	☐	Pretends
☐	☐	Reasons, negotiates and bargains
☐	☐	Uses humour
☐	☐	Talks about own feelings
☐	☐	Enquires about others' feelings

Comments

_____

_____

_____

_____

_____

_____

Routledge
Taylor & Francis Group

COMMUNICATION DEVELOPMENT PROFILE QUESTIONNAIRE

Name [ ] **Date** [ ]

Completed by [ ]

Use of Communication Skills
what and why the child communicates

Established Communicators

Conversational skills: P6–P8

Conversations

Working within	Consistent level				
☐	☐	Initiating	☐	☐	Terminating
☐	☐	Maintaining	☐	☐	Repairing

Body language

☐	☐	Eye contact	☐	☐	Fidgeting
☐	☐	Facial expression	☐	☐	Distance
☐	☐	Posture			

How you talk

☐	☐	Volume	☐	☐	Tone
☐	☐	Speed	☐	☐	Intelligibility
☐	☐	Fluency			

Awareness

☐	☐	Awareness of the listener's needs

Comments

_____

_____

_____

_____

_____

_____

COMMUNICATION DEVELOPMENT PROFILE QUESTIONNAIRE

Name [   ] **Date** [   ]

Completed by [   ]

Profile Summary & Aims

Summary of skills

Aims

COMMUNICATION DEVELOPMENT PROFILE QUESTIONNAIRE

Name [   ] **Date** [   ]

Completed by [   ]

Continuation Sheet

(Copy this sheet as many times as you need)

Routledge
Taylor & Francis Group
ROUTLEDGE

COMMUNICATION DEVELOPMENT PROFILE QUESTIONNAIRE

Name   Date

Completed by

Bibliography

Anderson-Wood L & Rae Smith B, 1997, *Working with Pragmatics: A Practical Guide to Promoting Communicative Confidence*, Speechmark, Bicester.

Bracken B, 1998, *Bracken Basic Concept Scale – Revised*, Harcourt Assessment, Oxford.

Buck D & Davis V, 2001, *Assessing Pupils' Performance using the P Levels,* Berger A (ed), David Fulton, London.

Bzoch KR & League R, 1970, 1999 (2nd edn), *The REEL (Receptive–Expressive Emergent Language) Scale*, Pro-ed, Texas.

Cavanna A, 2003, 'Materials for Courses', unpublished resource sheet, S&LT Department, South Devon Healthcare NHS Trust.

Child C, 2004, *Choices, Changes and Challenges*, S&LT Department, South Devon Healthcare NHS Trust.

Cooper J, Moodley M & Reynell J, 1978, *Helping Language Development. A developmental programme for children with early language handicaps*, Edward Arnold, London.

Coupe J, Barton L, Barber M, Collins L, Levy D & Murphy D, 1985, *The Affective Communication Assessment*, Melland School, Manchester.

Coupe O'Kane J & Goldbart J, 1998, *Communication Before Speech,* David Fulton, London.

Dewart H & Summers S, 1988, *The Pragmatics Profile of Early Communication Skills*, NFER-NELSON, Windsor.

Dewart H & Summers S, 1995, *The Pragmatics Profile of Everyday Communication Skills in School-Age Children*, NFER-NELSON, Windsor.

Gerard K, 1987, *Checklist for Communicative Competence*, Unpublished.

Grunwell P, 1982, *Clinical Phonology,* Croom Helm, London.

Johnson M, 2003, *Verbal Reasoning Skills Assessment,* S&LT Dept, Kent and Canterbury Hospital, East Kent Coastal Teaching PCT.

Kelly A, 1996, *Talkabout: A Social Communication Skills Package*, Speechmark, Bicester.

Kiernan G & Reid B, 1987, *The Pre-Verbal Communication Schedule (PVCS)*, NFER-NELSON, Windsor.

Knowles W & Masidlover M, 1982, *The Derbyshire Language Scheme*, Derbyshire County Council.

Millar S & Aitken S, 2003, *Personal Communication Passports: Guidelines for Good Practice*, Call Centre, University of Edinburgh.

Money D & Thurman S, 1994, 1996, *Talkabout Teaching Package,* Speechmark, Bicester.

Nind M & Hewett D, 2001, *A Practical Guide To Intensive Interaction*, BILD, Kidderminster.

QCA (Qualification and Curriculum Authority), 2001, *Planning, Teaching and Assessing the Curriculum for Pupils with Learning Disability*, QCA, London.

QCA, 2003, *The Foundation Stage Profile Handbook – Access to the Foundation Curriculum for Children with a Range of Special Needs*, QCA, London.

QCA, 2005, *Using the P-Scales*, QCA, London.

Rinaldi W, 1992a, *Social Use of Language Programme*, NFER-NELSON, Windsor.

Rinaldi W, 1992b, *Working with Language-Impaired Teenagers with Moderate Language Difficulties*, I CAN, London.

Stephenson J & Linfoot K, 1996, 'Intentional Communication and Graphic Symbol Use by Students with Severe Intellectual Disability', *International Journal of Disability, Development and Education* 43, pp147–65.

Tannock R, Girolametto L & Siegal L, 1992, 'Language Intervention with Children Who Have Developmental Delays: Effects of an Interactive Approach', *American Journal on Mental Retardation* 97, pp145–60.

Ware J, 1996, *Creating a Responsive Environment for People with Multiple Learning Difficulties*, David Fulton, London.

Woods G & Acors D, 1999, *PORIC (Personal Objects Representation Independence Consolidation: Method for Instructing Children in the Use of Concepts)*, Nutshell Services, Essex.

Useful Publications

The Hanen Centre produces a wide range of courses and publications which focus on the development of children's communication and language skills through adult–child interaction.

Further details can be obtained from:
>The Hanen Centre
>Suite 515 – 1075 Bay Street
>Toronto
>Ontario
>Canada
>M5S 2B1
>tel: (001) 416 921-1073
>fax: (001) 416 921-1225
>email: info@hanen.org
>website: www.hanen.org

Useful Courses

'I CAN' provide information and training on a wide range of speech, language and communication issues.

Cummins K & Hulme S, *Parent–Child Interaction,* I CAN Course.

This useful publication is available as part of an I CAN course on parent–child interaction.

Further information can be obtained from:
>I CAN
>4, Dyers Building
>Holborn
>London
>EC1N 2QP
>tel: 0845 225 4071
>website: www.ican.org.uk